HIV/AIDS IN SUB-SAHARAN AFRICA

Understanding the Implications of Culture & Context

HIV/AIDS

IN SUB-SAHARAN AFRICA

UNDERSTANDING THE IMPLICATIONS OF CULTURE & CONTEXT

EDITORS
JEAN BAXEN & ANDERS BREIDLID

UCT
PRESS

HIV/AIDS in Sub-Saharan Africa: Understanding the Implications of Culture & Context

First published 2009

UCT Press
an imprint of
Juta & Company Ltd
Mercury Crescent
Wetton, 7780
Cape Town, South Africa

ISBN 978-1-91989-518-5

Project managed by Marlinee Chetty
Production co-ordinator: Charles Mackriel
Editing by Alex Potter
Proofreading by Karoline Hanks
Indexing by Ethné Clarke
Typeset by ANdtp Services
Cover designed by Jacques Nel
Printed and bound by Shumani Printers

Typeset in Helvetica Neue 9.5pt on 12pt

This book has been peer reviewd by critical readers.

Table of Contents

Contributors

Bernice Adonis obtained her Higher Diploma in Education at Hewat College of Education, a BEd (Honours) in 2002 and her MEd in 2006 from the University of Cape Town (UCT). She is currently employed as a lecturer at False Bay College in Cape Town, South Africa.

Jean Baxen is Associate Professor at the Faculty of Education, Rhodes University. She was Senior Lecturer in the School of Education at the University of Cape Town for the duration of the project that resulted in this book. Here she taught courses on social identity and HIV/AIDS, research methodology, diversity in education and contemporary policy reform.She has also worked as a teacher, curriculum developer, researcher and consultant on curriculum and HIV/AIDS.

Anders Breidlid is Professor of International Education at Oslo University College, Norway, and has conducted research in South Africa, Sudan, Cuba and Chile. He headed, with Jean Baxen, a research project funded jointly by the National Research Foundation and Norway Research Council on Schooling, Cultural Values, HIV/AIDS and Education. He has been a visiting professor at UCT (1997–98); the Instituto Pedagogico Latinamericano y Caribeno, Havana (2005); and the Pontifica Universidad Catolica, Santiago/Villarrica (2008–09).

Aysha Hattas obtained her Diploma in Education in 1990 and Higher Diploma in Education in 1995 at Hewat College of Education, and a BEd (Hons) in 2002 and MEd in 2006 at UCT. She was a part-time lecturer on the course Philosophy of Care and Health Promotion in the Public Health Department at the University of the Western Cape. She currently lectures at the Cape Peninsula University of Technology. Her areas of specialisation are Life Orientation, HIV/AIDS, research and literacy.

Mamatsoso Matsoso-Makhate completed her undergraduate studies at the University of Lesotho. She went on to complete her BEd (Hons) and MEd at UCT, where she joined the project that led to the contribution in this book. She is a high school teacher in Lesotho.

Julia Kate Nupen completed her post-graduate studies at UCT. She taught for a few years and also lectured part-time in the School of Education at UCT. She is currently employed as the Human Resource Development Facilitator at Truworths head office in Cape Town.

Marit Petersen is a teacher by profession and she has been employed as a primary school teacher for several years in Oslo, Norway. She completed her MPhil in Multicultural and International Education at Oslo University College in 2007. She currently lectures at the Centre for Adult Education (Bærum Kommune Voksenopplæringssenter-BKVO) in Bærum, Norway.

Hilda Rolls completed a three-year Primary Teacher's Diploma at Hewat Training College in 1982, the Higher Diploma in Education through the Western Cape College of Education in 1997, and a BEd (Hons) in 2003 and MEd in 2005 at UCT. She currently teaches at Erica Primary School, where she has served for the past 23 years.

Gerald Wangenge-Ouma is a post-doctoral fellow and co-ordinator of the MEd (Higher Education Studies) programme at the University of the Western Cape. He was awarded a PhD by UCT in June 2007. He is a recipient of several research fellowships and has published in diverse areas, including schooling, HIV/AIDS and the youth, and higher education policy. Recent publications include articles in *Higher Education*, *The Journal of Higher Education Policy and Management*, and *The South African Journal of Higher Education.*

Acknowledgements

We are indebted to the National Research Foundation of South Africa and the Norway Research Council for funding the project on Schooling, Cultural Values and HIV/AIDS from 2002 to 2006 that resulted in peer-reviewed articles and the completion of six master's dissertations and a doctoral thesis. This project gave impetus to this book, with each researcher contributing directly or indirectly to its contents. We are grateful to the students who worked tirelessly to make the project a success.

This project would not have been a success without the willing participation of the schools, teachers and learners referred to in the book. Sincere thanks to those at each participating school.

Heartfelt thanks to Gerald Wangenge-Ouma, who is not only a contributor, but also edited earlier draft chapters. The book was reviewed by Prof. Crain Soudien, School of Education, UCT and Dr Halla Holmarsdottir, Oslo University College. Thank you for your insightful comments and for believing in the project.

Finally, special thanks to our respective families who were not only supportive, but also endlessly patient and willing to put up with our demanding schedules. We are also grateful to friends who unknowingly supported us.

Foreword

How does one make sense of the significance of the HIV/AIDS pandemic in South Africa? How does one take the disease and its accompanying afflictions and begin to understand what impact it has on the lives of ordinary people as they make their way through the rituals and everyday regularities of their worlds? How does one come to terms with the awful reality that life expectancy rates for South African males are now lower than they might have been a hundred years ago? How, more pertinently for the purposes of this book, does one begin to mediate the complex meaning of the HIV/AIDS pandemic, not just as a medical phenomenon, but as a social experience that is changing how people live, form relationships and dream dreams for themselves? How do people in education even begin to explain for themselves and for the young people they teach, in schools and universities, the deep significance of this extraordinary development in the life of the country?

Clearly, ordinary people — even people who have had the privilege of education — are struggling to come to terms with what HIV/AIDS means for them. The virtue of this book is that it provides one of the first South African responses to this challenge. It brings together the collaborative work of a number of South African and Norwegian researchers who went into communities and schools across the country to hear what children, young people, teachers and policy makers were saying about their encounters with the disease. Furthermore, it attempts to make sense of these voices in terms that are neither naive nor disrespectful. What does this mean? Apart from the innovativeness of this work and the degree to which its contributors have approached no-go areas such as child sexuality, and religion and sexuality, which are of themselves significant, what the book is doing is putting together a body of discussion that fundamentally shifts the centre of gravity in the HIV/AIDS and education discussion. The nature of this shift is essentially about moving from the didactic and normative model, which is currently dominant, to an approach that is saying that those talking about and mediating the disease need to come to terms with its sociological complexity.

All the contributions in the book are focused on the sociological complexity surrounding the disease. The book will no doubt be controversial. Many may find it too daring, too sweeping in its assessment of what is going on in communities, or even too broad in the way in which the complexity is experienced. The fact that it will do this is, however, its strength. Hopefully, what debate, or even debates, around this complexity will stimulate, is a sense that things are not what they seem. The incapacitating problem that is being experienced around the significance of the disease, and particularly in the communities where it is exacting such a heavy toll, is the deep anxiety that people feel when they try to talk about what it is that they are going through. Too often, the words and frameworks that are being drawn on to deal with it are those of previous problems and previous experiences. The fact of the matter is that the world as people know it has been ruptured by the disease, which is rearticulating the meaning of love, sex, kinship, comradeliness and, crucially, life and death. Things are not what they seem. A book like this has the potential to help make the point that important things — who we are and how we stand in relation to each other — have been altered by the disease.

Presenting the book as a provocation is, of course, assuming a position of being in the knowing, of having something that other people do not have, but ought to have. This is always the danger of being an academic. The approach that the contributors have taken to this text has, however, been one of respect. They have not taken their privileged positions of advantage for granted. In the process, they have begun to understand — and this is a lesson that they keep having to confront — that the privilege they have acquired brings with it major responsibility. The book they offer is fulfilling part of that responsibility. It is about placing into the public domain insight into the complexity of the social experience that HIV/AIDS constitutes.

I am thankful to Jean Baxen and Anders Breidlid for the opportunity to be a small part of their project. I would like to say to them that this work makes an important contribution to that larger project of understanding the place of South Africa in the world and the immense potential South Africa has of teaching the world what it means to be human in conditions of such intense difference. This is difference not only of the obvious kind — race, class and gender — but difference of the kind that also recognises distinctions between the well and the unwell; the safe and the unsafe. We who conduct our lives as scholars in South Africa have the perverse privilege of sitting in the front row of one of the great dramas of the human experiment. Many of us handle this privilege as voyeurs and derive from the pain and misery we see only a narrow kind of self-serving value. May we always be much more than this. May we come to this challenge with a sense that as we learn and dare to speak in new ways — ways that actually shift the nature of popular conversation — we never forget that the scholarly project is fundamentally about the public good.

Crain Soudien
Professor, School of Education at UCT

December 2008

The book is dedicated to those teachers for whom teaching about the pandemic is a way of being rather than an act of duty.

Introduction

This book is the result of a research project in South Africa on how the HIV/AIDS pandemic is perceived by various stakeholders in a South African context. The study suggests that it is important to focus on how and where the production and reproduction of HIV/AIDS discourse takes place. The reason for this is that the 'how' and 'where' shape and give character to individual and collective responses to HIV/AIDS, but are also, critically in this book, implicated in the ways in which both individuals and groups make their identities. The book, therefore, highlights the social and cultural practices shaping communities' responses to and uptake of the pandemic. Using a variety of social theory approaches, it analyses various contexts in which discourse production about HIV/AIDS takes place and shows how various stakeholders respond to and reproduce the various resulting discourses in different ways. By exploring the complex and sometimes contradictory spaces where HIV/AIDS discourses are negotiated, the book's chapters present a picture of the HIV/AIDS problematic that transcends the current simplistic approaches to the pandemic that often emphasise the need for a more knowledgeable populace.

It emerged very early on in the project that any exploration of HIV/AIDS needed to take account of its interrelatedness with sex, sexuality and disease, and ways in which the pandemic was embedded in these discourses. Thus, chapters are not limited to experiences of the pandemic. Rather, some explore identity construction in the context of HIV/AIDS, foregrounding how the dominant discourses of gender, sexuality and disease act as dominant mediatory tools that communities draw on to understand, interpret and make meaning of their individual and collective identities.

The book is therefore as much about identity construction as it is about HIV/AIDS. It explores how a pandemic of this nature offers different possibilities for making the self, amid constraints imposed by dominant structures and discourses. Some chapters highlight the tension between modernity and tradition, while others illustrate how this becomes a resource for the shaping of new identities. Other chapters show how positions are taken up either to maintain or protect a 'fixed' identity. The outcome is a book that demonstrates the complexity of the relationship between identity and context.

A distinguishing feature of the book is that all the chapters are based on data collected from the same seven communities. A point of difference among chapters is either in the emphasis on primary or secondary school sites, or the population sourced. Methods for conducting the study included interviews, and observational and survey data. The overarching aim in collecting data was to solicit experiences, views and perspectives across the seven community sites that could provide material for a sociocultural understanding of how the pandemic manifests itself as a social phenomenon. An additional aim was to develop a research landscape for the project that would include a variety of research sites (churches, schools, mosques, homes and tabernacles) and respondents (religious leaders, school heads, teachers, children and youth) as well as a spread of socioeconomic and sociocultural contexts in which research was carried out. Chapters in this book thus emphasise the need to go beyond asking questions about what knowledge people in different communities hold about the pandemic to asking questions about how they make meaning of their individual and collective identities in a context riven with multiple and often contradictory messages about HIV/AIDS.

Methodologically, this book proposes a shift away from quantitative knowledge, attitudes and practice-related studies that seek to investigate the knowledge base of members of different population groups to approaches that emphasise views and experiences from an insider perspective. It examines experiences of those living and working in the context of HIV/AIDS and, through the use of qualitative methodologies that take into account the sensitivity and stigmatisation of the topic, seeks to shed light on aspects of the pandemic that need to be taken into account if interventions at all levels are to prove effective. The book shifts the discourse away from an emphasis on medical and catastrophic discourses and suggests a more hermeneutic approach to researching HIV/AIDS that addresses the contexts in which people make meaning of their lives in relation to the pandemic.

Data collection was confined to communities in the Western Cape Province of South Africa. Permission to conduct the research was given by the Research Unit of the Western Cape Education Department.

Sites were identified through random and purposive sampling strategies. This included selecting primary and secondary schools representing different communities. Two steps were followed in this process of selection. Firstly, and in order to select communities, all primary and secondary schools in the Cape Metropole were grouped according to the racial categories used during the period of apartheid to determine the school and geographic locations of the respective communities. This involved categorising schools using the racial categories of black, white, coloured and Indian. These were further divided into secondary and primary schools. Once the step of racial categorisation was complete, schools were then randomly selected within each category and school level. Additional schools were selected in the coloured and black categories. Since there are only four Indian schools in the Western Cape, only one was included in the research.

One of the primary aims of the project was to gain insight into the views of, responses to and experiences of the pandemic of different communities. It made sense, therefore, to include more communities hardest hit by the HIV/AIDS, hence the skewed number of schools per racial group. It has to be noted that 23 white primary schools were approached to participate in the study. None was available, citing busy schedules as the primary reason for non-participation. Table 1 shows the final number of schools in each racial category.

Table 1: Racial categorisation and number of schools

Racial category	Number of schools	
	Secondary	*Primary*
Coloured	2	2
Indian	0	1
Black	2	3
White	1	0

Once schools were identified, letters seeking permission to use each selected school in the research project were sent out. School visits were thereafter conducted to hold discussions with the school management team and staff. These discussions highlighted the broad project aims and objectives. Importantly, though, each investigator sought additional permission from his/her respective respondents, who signed letters of consent each time.

The book is divided into four parts.

In part 1, the editors set the scene for a sociological reading of the HIV/AIDS landscape by exploring the limitations in the educational research agenda. Claiming that research in HIV/AIDS is predominantly based on the disciplines of economics, medicine and epidemiology, Baxen and Breidlid call for research that takes account of the cultural and social context in which meanings and interpretations of HIV/AIDS are rooted, produced and reproduced. This, they argue, would allow for a more nuanced reading of the articulation between knowledge and practice.

Underlining that the disease is as much social as it is biomedical, the editors call for differentiated interventions that take cognisance of how cultural and contextual factors shape responses to and interpretations of the pandemic, which in their view seem to fuel the pandemic.

In part II, two such contexts in relation to HIV/AIDS are explored, namely the school context and the religious context. In chapter 4, Bernice Adonis with Jean Baxen examine school culture and discuss how it acts as a filter to the knowledge taught about HIV/AIDS. According to their findings, school culture is important in the mediation of knowledge and information about HIV/AIDS, as it influences what and how teachers teach and, more importantly, how teachers position themselves in relation to the content of their lessons. Teachers whose beliefs and values were similar to those of the school, and who lived in close proximity to the school, seemed to align themselves and the school's culture with their respective communities' practices, thereby entrenching these practices and thus making it difficult to insert a different discourse from the dominant one. Teachers were restrained when their values and those of the school were different. For the most part, teachers suppressed their personal positions and complied with the culture of the school. This, Adonis and Baxen argue, offers little agency for teachers to work outside the 'acceptable' discourse for fear of the personal and professional consequences.

Aysha Hattas' focus in chapter 5 is on religious leaders and their responses to HIV/AIDS. In particular, she examines their attitudes to sex and sexual behaviour in relation to the HIV/AIDS pandemic. While the study is not representative of the opinions of the religious leaders in toto in the Cape Town area, it reveals how within this multi-faith group of religious leaders, two types of discourses emerge. The first — what Hattas refers to as a 'closed' discourse — is one that adheres to more traditional religious principles, and within it, leaders are unwilling to acknowledge the existence of HIV/AIDS in their communities. The 'closed' discourse is resistant to change and does not allow for any religious adjustment to address the pandemic, viewing condom use, for example, as not only unacceptable, but actually immoral. The 'open' discourse, while still adhering to basic religious principles, acknowledges the changing context of religious beliefs and allows for modern interpretations and choice. In contrast to the 'closed' discourse, the 'open' one addresses the challenges people face in the wake of HIV/AIDS and thus creates a window of opportunity for addressing critical issues that militate against behaviour change and the deceleration of the pandemic.

Part III begins with Hilda Rolls' chapter 6, which explores how primary school children construct their sexual identities. She argues that children's sexual identity construction is context specific and situational, and illustrates how games, chores and entertainment act as discursive spaces for sexual identity construction. Children, she proposes, position themselves in particular ways, meaning that engagement in these social activities supports the shaping of masculine and feminine identities. According to Rolls, parents and siblings are important role models who contribute to sexual identity construction and, by implication, either reproduce or rupture dominant constructions. She acknowledges the dominance of heterosexuality and describes the difficulty and challenges one learner faced in not subscribing to the dominant biological construction of gender. Children's sexuality cannot, according to Rolls, be viewed as a separate entity, but must be viewed as an integrated process where the children continually construct and deconstruct their sexual experiences in interaction with significant others.

Mamatsoso Matsoso-Makhate with Gerald Wangenge-Ouma analyse factors shaping secondary school learners' sexual identity construction in chapter 7. According to their findings, the students 'perform' as opposed to 'are' their gendered roles. They reproduce dominant practices where males are perceived as 'initiators' and females as the 'pursued', even in circumstances that allow for the subversion of such roles. Matsoso-Makhate and Wangenge-Ouma put forward the argument, though, that dichotomising feminine and masculine roles obscures the complex ways in which the traditional gendered discourse is both maintained and subverted. According to them, heterosexuality was the discourse from and through which boys, and particularly girls, made their sexual selves. While girls both maintained and subverted the dominant discourse by using networks in initiating relationships, in performing their 'expected' gendered roles they almost always gave boys the power to make the choice of whether or not to pursue a relationship. Thus boys, somewhat paradoxically, still maintained the role of initiator, leaving little room for girls to make different choices or reproduce a different discourse. Boys, the researchers found, adopted a taken-for-granted orientation to their sexual identity construction. It was the girls who often complied with 'expected' practice, leaving boys to continue their actions unaltered and unquestioned. The fact that particularly the girls performed their 'expected' gendered roles has far-reaching implications, especially in the context of HIV/AIDS, as it undermines the girls' agency.

In chapter 8, Julia Nupen with Gerald Wangenge-Ouma analyses young people's perceptions and understandings of risk in the context of HIV/AIDS. Their findings point to many young people having unrealistic conceptions of invincibility and invulnerability with regard to HIV infection, even in the face of experience of the disease through relatives and friends. These conceptions influence how these young people make relationship choices and their participation in risky sexual behaviours. The way young people make sexual choices and their thoughts about risk in relation to HIV/AIDS are integrally linked to the context in which they construct their sexual identities and make meaning of their lives. This, as the authors find, is always in relation to the 'other'. Their chapter points to the importance of context and how it always acts as a frame of reference for constructing sexual identity. This context is volatile and offers many possibilities for making different sexual identities. However, while this might be so, the authors found that this context is also regulated by dominant discourses that disallow a different uptake of sexual identities. The authors maintain that understanding the ways in which context shapes and is shaped by those who inhabit the spaces is important in understanding both the risk factor in relation to HIV infection and the implication this has for designing effective interventions.

Following along the same vein as the other chapters in this section, Marit Petersen in chapter 9 examines the ways in which young women in particular interpret and enact gender roles within sexual relationships. By exploring how gender dynamics influence sexual choices among adolescents in two different settings (one predominantly black and the other a mixture of coloured and white) in the Cape Town area, Petersen finds that those adolescents in the predominantly black and poor setting are open to particular susceptibility that is encouraged by the way they position themselves in relation to hegemonic masculinities, patriarchy and 'expected' gender roles. She finds that, more often than not, these female adolescents complied with what she describes as a 'closed' hegemonic script. The coloured and white youth from the more affluent setting were better able not only to make different choices, but also to articulate these choices in situations where gender equity was more acceptable. Petersen calls this the 'open' script, which allows for different possibilities in making a sexual identity. Importantly, though, choices were available in both settings. However, those in the poor, predominantly black setting were more aware of the consequences of non-compliance, while youth in the more affluent setting seemed naive about the consequences their choices might have in relation to HIV infection and risk. Both groups were under risk, but for very different reasons. Like those of Matsoso-Makhate and Wangenge-Ouma, Petersen's findings point to the importance of understanding ways in which location shapes and is shaped by the actors and how this often reproduces practices that offer limited possibilities for particularly women to act differently or make choices that ensure their sexual well-being.

Jean Baxen and Anders Breidlid

PART 1

LIMITATIONS IN THE EDUCATIONAL RESEARCH AGENDA

(1994–2005)

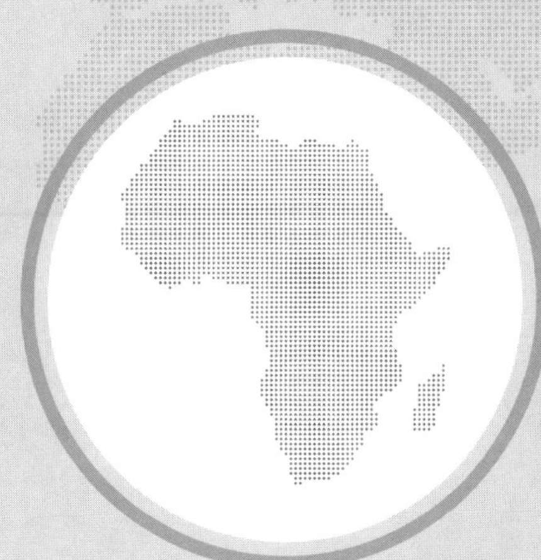

SUB-SAHARAN AFRICA

Chapter 1

Jean Baxen
University of Cape Town

Anders Breidlid
Oslo University College

Researching HIV/AIDS and Education in Sub-Saharan Africa: Examining the Gaps and Challenges[1]

Introduction

In this chapter, we argue that research in HIV/AIDS within the education sector is largely influenced by dominant discourses within the economics, medicine and epidemiology sectors that, by and large, fail to take into consideration the social and cultural embeddedness of the disease. Through a critique of the research conducted in the last ten years, we trace three major trends of research in HIV/AIDS and education and suggest that these, while useful, neglect the situated context in which messages, knowledge, experience and practice are produced, reproduced and expressed. We suggest that current research has to pay close attention to developing an understanding of where and how knowledge is produced and reproduced if the education sector is to contribute to enabling teachers and learners to make informed choices about their behavioural practices. This chapter forms the basis for what follows in the rest of the book.

While the health and economic sectors in many countries where HIV/AIDS has been prevalent seem to have recognised and explored the impact of this pandemic on their respective sectors for some time now, sectors such as education and social services have remained peripheral to the debates until very recently (Johnson, 2000). This seems partly due to the relatively low number of people dying of HIV/AIDS in comparison to those infected. The upshot is that even though much has been written about the projected impact of HIV/AIDS on the education sector (Coombe, 2000a; 2001; Johnson, 2000; Kelly, 2000; Barnett & Whiteside, 2002), the effect of the pandemic on this sector as a whole is only beginning to enter research debates. There is a growing acceptance that a key strategy in combating the pandemic involves an intersectoral approach that draws on health, education and social welfare systems and structures (Coombe, 2000a). Notwithstanding this, education, as Kelly suggests, 'might be the single most powerful weapon against HIV transmission' (Kelly, 2000:9), since through it potential messages that can lead to a change in sexual behaviour are transmitted.

On one level, researchers around the world agree with Kelly, since much has been written about the perceived efficacy of education programmes and how education, particularly formal schooling, might be one of the key preventive strategies against the virus (Kelly, 2002; Coombe, 2000a). The underlying assumption that these authors make

1 An earlier version of this chapter has appeared in the *Journal of Education* (34, 2004, 9–29). The authors are grateful for permission to reprint here.

is that schools have a 'captive' audience, ie children, many of whom, it is assumed, may not be sexually active. The assumption, too, is that providing children with sufficient knowledge may serve to delay their sexual debut and enable them to make informed decisions about their sexual practices and behaviours. In this chapter we explore how and in what way current educational research has facilitated a better understanding of schooling, teaching and learning about HIV/AIDS. In short, we explore what is/has been the educational research agenda, how it is shaped and what the underlying assumptions are of the research questions posed. Moreover, we focus on what has been researched and how the research in education has contributed to and extended the debates about HIV/AIDS. Finally, the chapter seeks to highlight the gaps in the research through an analysis of the kind of educational research conducted in the last decade nationally and internationally on HIV/AIDS and education.

In particular, this chapter uses the issues raised above as the catalyst for a critique of the focus and nature of research carried out within the educational sector. It argues that this research, particularly within a South African context, is limited in scope because the context in which HIV/AIDS-related processes take place, as a discursive field (which includes social and cultural practices), is either absent or unaccounted for in many of the studies under scrutiny. This becomes apparent when two critical considerations are taken into account: the changing nature of the disease and its major effect on Third World populations such as those in sub-Saharan Africa, where prevalence is among the highest in the world. Briefly, what makes this pandemic different in this particular context is its prevalence among heterosexual communities, a phenomenon not as ubiquitous in First World contexts (even though there might be a growing number of reported cases in the latter contexts). This shift in prevalence brings with it new challenges of how the disease is perceived, experienced, understood, responded to and researched among different groups within and across communities. What then seems necessary are different sets of questions that extend the debate beyond *what we know* about the disease to *how we come to know what we perceive we know*. In its argument, the chapter postulates that one way of refocusing the agenda is by interrogating the underlying assumptions of the research on HIV/AIDS and by examining *what* research is conducted, *how* research is conducted and by *whom*, using *which* methodological lenses. The field of education, the chapter argues, can contribute meaningfully to understanding the discursive fields of practice in which messages and knowledge about the pandemic are articulated, produced and reproduced by not merely reproducing forms of research that respond to *what* we come to know, but rather *how* or *whether* we *can* come to know. This includes raising questions about the nature and focus of research in educational contexts.

Research needs to pay close attention to *where* and *how* the production and reproduction of the HIV/AIDS discourse takes place. This discourse should be understood within deeply embedded *situated, discursive spaces* (contexts) where social and cultural practices are negotiated, produced and reproduced. Within such spaces, the linearity of knowledge and behavioural practices cannot be assumed. Significant to this discussion is a consideration of these spaces as negotiated and complex, sometimes contradictory and conflictual, but always in the process of changing, thereby making messages not always easily reproducible. Through a brief review of the nature of research on HIV/AIDS in educational settings, the next section of the chapter provides a quick glimpse into the current research landscape. In a critical discussion, the final section provides a rationale for considering context and culture as key elements in understanding the discourse of HIV/AIDS and schooling.

Research in education: Where is 'the gaze'?

Within the last decade, the majority of studies within education contexts may be categorised as falling within three broad areas of research, namely: *projective, KAP-type* (knowledge, attitude and practice) and *impact studies.* While the contexts (primarily limited to geographic site), target groups and sites may have differed, the fundamental research questions posed seemed to be shaped by a need to answer the question 'what' is known and perceived by various target groups, with little attention to 'how' they come to know, and 'where' (discursively) the knowledge they have is produced and reproduced. Through a brief analysis of each broad area of research in education, the perceived omissions, gaps and challenges are outlined below.

Projective studies within sub-Saharan contexts

Several studies commissioned in the last ten years (eg Johnson, 2000; World Bank, 2000) indicate that little is known about the effects of the pandemic on the various components of the education sector, particularly in Third World contexts. This is partly due to the lack of research in this field, but also due to policies that, while protecting the rights of the individual, on the one hand, serve to disadvantage the very persons they propose to protect, on the other. The studies, many of which are based on projections, do, however, provide a broad framework for understanding the projected impact this pandemic will have on the education sector. One such study is that conducted by Johnson (2000), who suggests that the education sector firstly needs to acknowledge that HIV/AIDS education is not only about ensuring good life skills and other prevention programmes; rather, it has to recognise that a significant percentage of the teaching corps will become ill and die. He warns that learner numbers will at first escalate, but thereafter decline due to either illness or home circumstances. By using customised projections of levels of infection and illness, Johnson intimates that HIV/AIDS will magnify the existing social and health problems experienced within the education sector. Not only will schools have to deal with aspects such as absenteeism by teachers, but also with children who are affected, infected and orphaned as a result of the pandemic. According to Johnson (2000), schools will need to be involved in identifying vulnerable children and finding ways to enable such children to cope under severe circumstances. Cohen (2002) seems to support Johnson by suggesting that the impact of HIV/AIDS in education is primarily related to the decimation of personnel, but nevertheless argues that there is insufficient data to make reliable projections.

HIV/AIDS will affect education through a

> reduction in demand and supply, reduction in availability of resources, adjustments in response to the special needs of a rapidly increasing number of orphans, adaptation to new interactions both within schools and between schools and communities, curriculum modifications, altered roles that have to be adopted by teachers and the education system, the ways in which schools and the education system are organised, the planning and management of the system, and the donor support for education (Kelly, 2000:1).

Like M. J. Kelly (2000), Akoulouze, Rugalema and Khanye (2001) note that due to HIV/AIDS:

- there will be less and less demand for education, as orphans (especially girls) leave school;
- teachers will also leave the education system due to their own ill health or the need to look after others; and
- education departments will not be able to make reliable predictions about future needs. The departments will also suffer personnel losses in administration, management and support areas.

In a similar vein, Coombe (2000a) describes how the education sector in South Africa might manage the impact of HIV/AIDS. Her study cites teachers as one of the population groups especially at risk, because they are 'educated, mobile and relatively affluent' (Coombe, 2000a:15). As part of the response strategy, she suggests a multisectoral approach to the pandemic that moves the focus away from viewing HIV/AIDS as a health problem to one that acknowledges that it is a social and institutional problem. She proposes that one area of focus should be on enabling teachers to gain a better understanding of the way in which HIV/AIDS will impact on their professional lives. The proposal is that teachers should also be made aware of how other sectors are losing staff that will need to be replaced. Moreover, attention must be paid to developing strategies that will respond to the pandemic in creative ways. These strategies, it is suggested, will need to consider, among other things, training replacement personnel (Coombe, 2000a). While emerging research in sub-Saharan Africa, particularly in South Africa (eg Education Labour Relations Council, 2005a), gives some indication of the pandemic's effects, this is still insufficient to measure its full material effects on schools and school communities.

The accuracy of the projections described above is not under discussion here. The contribution these studies make is useful in as much as they provide a broad overview of the potential problem that education sectors might experience at the systemic level in the face of the pandemic. In this regard, they have been invaluable in drawing attention to the need for a proactive response and some strategic planning within education ministries. These studies, notwithstanding, have not addressed — and were not intended to address — what is actually happening at the chalk face, in schools and classrooms or within communities seriously affected by morbidity and mortality due to the pandemic. Their contribution has been, by and large, at a policy and advocacy level, forcing some recognition of the need for action within the education ministries, on the one hand, and the need for further research (on schools, teachers, learners and such like), on the other hand, which the next category of studies attempts to address.

KAP studies on HIV/AIDS

Within this category, studies (eg Wood, Maepa & Jewkes, 1997; Levine & Ross, 2002; Varga, 1997; Pettifor et al, 2004; Kalichman et al, 2005) have sought to examine and gain some understanding of *what* knowledge, attitudes and practices (KAP) those participating in the educational endeavour (teachers, youth, adolescents, and so on) have. Often these studies have as their main outcome recommendations for the development of 'effective' prevention strategies for those perceived as 'most vulnerable' (in many instances, adolescents and youth between the ages of 14 and 24). This trend of researching through KAP studies is consistent with earlier research carried out within the medical, health and social welfare sectors, which have a longer history of researching the pandemic. In the field of education, what these studies assume is a correlation between knowledge and behaviour, since the primary aim of such studies (and the use of results) has been to contribute to the development of 'more effective' prevention programmes. The upshot, as will be evident in the next section, is a delinking of the individual from context and culture and a downplaying of the discursive nature of the pandemic and the cultural and social practices in which it is embedded. There is also a presupposition about children in primary schools as being asexual, which leads to the assumption that mostly high school children should be the target of research and intervention programmes. Another assumption is that teachers are able to and will teach about deeply private, personal topics in a public space. In so doing, they bring their own sexuality and sexual practises into the spotlight. It is also assumed that the content (eg the biological nature of the disease) of research is uncontested; the dislocation of sexual identity from cultural and social discourse; the disconnection of sexual identity from larger debates about power and gender; and finally, inferences about the uncontested nature of the research process.

Youth and HIV/AIDS

The focus in research on youth and HIV/AIDS has, by and large, been on knowledge about the disease and the relation between knowledge and reproductive health. An emerging body of research concentrating on sociocultural contexts forms the second strand of research in this section.

Knowledge of HIV/AIDS and reproductive health

There is very little co-ordinated information on what South African youth know about reproductive health. Judging from some of the studies, some South African youth have a very sketchy understanding of reproduction, puberty and sexually transmitted diseases (Wood et al, 1997). This study found that teenagers had very little sexual knowledge prior to and during the first few months of sexual activity, including not being aware that intercourse can result in pregnancy. Similar conclusions were drawn by Harrison et al (2001), who found that girls in KwaZulu-Natal had poor factual knowledge of sex. Such misinformation included cultural myths that reinforced beliefs that evil spirits would eat them if there was a delayed sexual debut. A further aspect of cultural myth was that boys would experience pain later if they did not have sex while they were young; also, boys who did not have sex while still young would accumulate sperm and be more likely to impregnate a girl later. Levine and Ross (2002) investigated the knowledge and attitudes towards AIDS of undergraduate university students. They found that although students had knowledge of the sexual transmission of AIDS, they did not report knowledge of vertical transmission. However, this trend seems to be changing in some communities. In a study commissioned by the Department of Health, Kelly (2000) found that youth had good access to accurate HIV/AIDS information and were regularly exposed to such information. This is confirmed by studies such as those by Pettifor et al (2004).

Socioeconomic and cultural constraints

As has already been suggested, young people are particularly vulnerable to HIV infection, with most HIV infection occurring among this group (Rivers & Aggleton, 1999; LeClerc-Madlala, 2002a). They do, however, face a great many problems in protecting their sexual and reproductive health, partly as a consequence of external pressures (socioeconomic and cultural) within the contexts they find themselves in, and partly as a result of how adolescence is commonly constructed, ie as a time of high risk and low responsibility. While in more traditional societies, sex education was offered by the community, this practice is no longer widespread or common, in part due to rapid urbanisation and migration disrupting community networks (Rivers & Aggleton, 1999). In more recent times, the tendency is for youth to receive information from peers and the media (Rivers & Aggleton, 1999), with girls often not being the target of information campaigns. During this period, it seems that adults are less certain of their roles than in the past, with teachers feeling particularly vulnerable in this regard. In many countries, teachers have reportedly complained of being embarrassed and ill-prepared to talk about sex with children. Here the very fluidity between the traditional and the modern may leave both adults and young people feeling marooned. Cohen (2002) describes the context of education programmes, and includes school environments that are not safe or health affirming, huge gaps between home and school, poverty and its often concomitant fatalism, disempowered women and images of masculinity that include promiscuity. Other studies confirm that the socioeconomic and cultural factors are major constraints in effecting behavioural sexual changes. These factors include the exchange of sex for material compensation (Rivers & Aggleton, 1999); alternative strategies for HIV protection; so-called cultural logic systems (Easton, 1999; Sobo, 1995); and class, education and religious affiliation as perceived protective mechanisms (Levine & Ross, 2002). Moreover, polygyny (the encouragement of multiple sexual partners), traditional medicine, repressive customary law and culturally defined control over women (Levine & Ross, 2002) all contribute to making efficient HIV protection more difficult. So, it would seem that even when readily available, 'knowledge' does not necessarily protect teenagers, because some South Africans are constructing their sexual identities and their safety from infection in terms of competing knowledge systems (Skinner, 2001) and within contexts that produce, reproduce and send conflicting messages to the youth.

Teachers and HIV/AIDS

At a systemic or macro-level, projections of how teachers are affected were discussed earlier. At a micro-level, teachers are affected by the HIV/AIDS pandemic in a number of ways. On one level they are, of course, affected by their students' infection, and by the spread of the disease in their communities. On another level, they themselves may be at risk of infection, or they may indeed be living with HIV/AIDS. They may also have infected family members whom they take care of. Notwithstanding the above, there is a marked lack of studies that focus research at the micro-level, and particularly on teachers and schools. In some studies where teachers have been subjects of research (eg Akoulouze et al, 2001), they have been positioned as deliverers of an uncontested, already negotiated body of HIV/AIDS knowledge within spaces (schools and institutions) that are unproblematic. In this regard, teachers have consequently been targets of training programmes that have largely portrayed them as lacking *knowledge and skills* to teach life skills or sex education programmes effectively. Other studies have attempted to describe teachers as more 'vulnerable' than the rest of society, citing reasons such as mobility as a key indicator (Kelly, 2002), this with the view to developing intervention programmes for them. Some (eg Bennel, 2003) have sought to negate this assumption by providing evidence that makes the argument of teacher vulnerability unsustainable.

Emerging work by the Education Labour Relations Council (2005a) in association with the Human Sciences Research Council, for example, shifts the spotlight back to systemic issues through a large-scale study of demand for and supply of teachers within South Africa. While such studies are important, and will indeed move the debate beyond a projection to what is actually happening at the chalk face, teachers as agents who act within conflicting discursive spaces are absent from the debate. Studies such as those of Buczekiewicz and Carnegie (2001) suggest that translating HIV knowledge into behaviour change means a change in how teachers teach. But, as they propose, it is sometimes difficult for teachers to reproduce the conditions of their training, and so equally difficult to reproduce the methods they were taught. In addition, these authors believe teachers need detailed guidance on content.

In addressing this gap, some work has emerged that begins to examine the relationship between teacher identity and teaching (eg Baxen, 2006; 2008). This work traces the complex relationship between teacher identity and classroom practice, showing how, amid supposedly adequate knowledge, teachers find it difficult to negotiate their way in life-skills classrooms when the topics of sexuality and HIV/AIDS are focused on.

Studies on intervention and training programmes

Many studies (suggested earlier in this paper) have confirmed that education is vital in the prevention of the spread of HIV/AIDS. For example, Kaufman and Stavros (2002) assert, by describing and assessing the impact of community resources (such as educational levels) on adolescent safe sex practices, that education has a powerful effect on the degree to which young people engage in risky sexual behaviour. Our findings suggest that schools have ample latitude to promote the knowledge, understanding and skills to enable young people to make responsible decisions about their sexual behaviour. They also suggest that educational effects may persist after school is completed, because the educational levels of other household members are found to have an important association with risky behaviour (Kaufman & Stavros, 2002).

Therefore, in finding ways to increase awareness of and suggest preventive measures against the disease, life-skills and sex education programmes have been developed within the formal school sector. These programmes have been aimed at providing children (in particular, the youth) with accurate information about the disease. Rivers and Aggleton (1999) note that the focus of school-based interventions is usually limited to youth in school, and the emphasis is usually on secondary schools as the target group. For instance, in South Africa, many sex education programmes are limited, but not exclusive, to secondary school learners as targets. This is despite research showing that interventions are most successful before the sexual debut (Rivers & Aggleton, 1999), on the one hand, and that primary schools are significant sites for the construction and reproduction of sexual identity among children (Renold, 2000; Wallis & VanEvery, 2000), on the other hand. The omission of such contextual realities, viewed against the backdrop of where HIV/AIDS prevalence is highest, namely in developing countries, where many people, especially girls, leave school after primary school and where the attendance of girl children is irregular (Rivers & Aggleton, 1999) and in some cases low, brings into sharp focus the limitation of such research foci (ie interventions at secondary schools). While there is no question that some intervention programmes have a notable degree of success in increasing knowledge, it cannot be assumed that this knowledge will lead to behaviour change (Grunseit & Aggleton, 1998). Indeed, a substantial literature review conducted by Grunseit and Aggleton (1998) shows that of the 53 studies reviewed, as many as 27 showed no effect on youth sexual practices. In an attempt to examine ways of increasing the possibility of behavioural change, Wight (1999) finds that learner-driven classes do not work as well as teacher-driven ones. Wight argues that there are severe limits to the efficacy of pupil empowerment in sex and HIV/AIDS education. Skinner (2001), however, finds that educators are seen as being out of touch with youth. He describes this as another factor distancing youth from scientific information and making them inclined to look to alternative sources of knowledge. Mirembe (2002), on the other hand, advocates learner involvement as a way of combating 'information fatigue' (see also Levine & Ross, 2002). She hypothesises that programmes would be more successful if learners were involved in devising and running them and suggests that there is a relationship between democratic classroom practice and programme success.

Context, culture and HIV/AIDS

Evident in the research, particularly in South Africa, is the untheorised manner in which constructs such as culture and the associated concept of cultural values are used, despite their employment in studies focusing on knowledge, attitude and behaviour regarding HIV/AIDS. A number of conceptual issues arise from the literature on cultural values, and on such values and HIV/AIDS. The first, and most important, is that the terms 'culture' or 'traditional culture' are often used to signify an essentialist African culture without careful definition of which African culture is being referred to. It is not clear in the South African research context to what extent the behaviour of Xhosa adolescents (Wood et al, 1997) can be compared with the behaviour of, for instance, Zulu adolescents (Tillotson & Maharaj, 2001). Of course, this is to some extent an indication of the South African problematic, where both the colonial and apartheid governments invested heavily in the idea of distinct cultural groups (Ntshoe, 1999; Fleisch, 1995). There is no discussion in the research reviewed of the fluidity of culture, either in terms of a continuum of 'traditional' and 'modern' behaviour, or in terms of relationships among different cultures, languages and ethnicities. Often in both apartheid and post-apartheid discourse, 'culture' is interpreted as a transcript for racial heritage. As such, researchers in the reviewed literature sometimes conflate language group and culture, explaining that, for example, the sample consists of Zulu-speaking South Africans, which may also indicate that the sample may be defined as of the Zulu culture.

In some studies, however, it may be inferred that the results are indicative of a specific culture's values (eg LeClerc-Madlala 2001a; 2001b; 2002a; Breidlid, 2002). What this brief discussion illustrates is that culture, particularly in the South African context, is a difficult term, and this may go some way to explaining the reluctance of researchers to engage directly with it in defining their sample or in theorising their results. While it is acknowledged that often tradition is subsumed in modern practices and vice versa, tension can exist where communities are still very traditional and youth are influenced by both tradition and modernity, thereby making difficult the challenge of navigating their way within social and cultural practices that are fluid and sometimes contradictory (Breidlid, 2002).

There are some indications that a more unified approach may be taken to South African values regarding HIV/AIDS. Wood and Jewkes (1997) completed a cross-racial project on the significance of adolescent gift giving to the dynamics of sexual decision making. Although their small focus group study found differences among the responses of different races, these may be characterised as differences of degree. Smith, Lucas and Latkin (1999) discuss social discourse as a factor in the efficacy of intervention programmes, noting that information about HIV/AIDS tends to be disseminated through rumour and gossip, and recommend that intervention programmes target social networks. This also opens up the possibility that culture should be thought of more broadly as groups associated by ways of communicating as well as (or even rather than) heritage. Although a number of South African studies acknowledge explicitly or implicitly the importance of cultural context in the efficacy of intervention programmes, few reviewed here have set out to study the influence of cultural belief on sexual negotiation and behaviour. In other words, although a number of studies *describe* South African cultural beliefs that have a bearing on sexual behaviour, the impact of cultural beliefs on sexual behaviour, negotiation and change is a matter of conjecture. Specifically, no studies reviewed here are investigations of the intersection between either cultural context or cultural beliefs and intervention programme efficacy. The reason for this may be the sensitivity of the issue due to issues of class, ethnicity and gender, and the possibility that focusing on culture may also be deemed politically incorrect in a nation striving to achieve a national identity across the former differences. One such example, however, is a study by Cohen (2002), who suggests that cultural aspects (besides socioeconomic circumstances) present serious constraints in the attempt to fight the pandemic. Similarly, Archie-Booker, Cervero and Langone (1999) suggest that HIV/AIDS prevention education must be responsive to culture in order to be effective and examine what prevents an intervention programme from being culturally relevant. Their results are a reminder that the generation and efficacy of culturally sensitive intervention programmes are not only matters of understanding the community, but of how the organisation offering the intervention operates. Few studies actively integrate the political or economic culture of the participants into the discussion, although these are also significant determinants of, for instance, how gender is constructed. Campbell and Mzaidume (2001) and Susser and Stein (2000) are examples of studies where economic and social differences within cultures are factored into the conceptual framework and (especially in the case of Susser and Stein) into the methodology. At the heart of the matter, however, seems to be the need for interrogating terms like 'culture' and 'cultural values' that are not only fundamental to the integrity of the research, but also to that of the efficacy of intervention programmes.

Discussion

Youth and HIV/AIDS

Evidenced in critiquing impact and intervention studies research carried out in sub-Saharan Africa and internationally is an emphasis on youth perceived either as vulnerable or sexually active, or, at the very least, sexually aware and therefore, by implication, a 'natural' target of prevention and intervention programmes. Underpinning these studies is an assumption too that these youth within the formal schooling sector are located primarily, if not exclusively, in *secondary* schools. These assumptions raise several key points. Firstly, the emphasis on intervention and prevention programmes (giving youth *more* knowledge) seems to be underpinned by reductionist views of the association between knowledge and behaviour. This view creates a dissociation of the interface among sexual identity, education and HIV/AIDS. More importantly, what it leaves unattended are the deeply complex nature of the social and cultural discursive fields in which youth receive and interpret the HIV/AIDS messages and how they understand, experience and use this knowledge in the face of or while constructing, performing and playing out their sexual identities. Particularly, *school* as one such *situated* discursive field that occupies a particular space in time is unaccounted for within this body of research. While some studies (eg LeClerc-Madlala, 2002a; Skinner, 2001) have begun to address this, the majority are still driven by the need to know 'what' knowledge youth have, with the view to providing them with 'more' knowledge, even in the face of its ineffectiveness. In addition, these studies do not account for the discursive social and cultural fields of practice where knowledge is not only produced, but also contested, negotiated, reproduced and embedded. While there is an emerging body of research that is beginning to consider the above, the fundamental methodological research question still seems to be driven by a medical discourse that does not give ascendancy to issues of gender, power and sexuality as deeply connected to constructions of safe sex, negotiation within relationships and HIV/AIDS knowledge. As LeClerc-Madlala (2002a) suggests, what is necessary in research about youth is a shift to understanding their construction of self and sexual identity, and how, in the face of HIV/AIDS, their vulnerability is exacerbated. Following this argument and critical to the discussion, disembedding cultural and social practices from the discursive *sites* in which these sexual identities are produced and reproduced seems to neglect primary schools as a 'key cultural arena for the production of sexuality and sexual identities' (Renold, 2000:309).

Teachers and HIV/AIDS

A stark omission within this body of research is work that considers teachers as producers, interpreters, reproducers, mediators and purveyors of knowledge and safe-sex messages, who work within discursive fields in which this knowledge is contested and may be considered secret and/or private. Where such gaps in research have been identified, the suggested response has been to examine ways of providing teachers with more information about HIV/AIDS, more training or more effective programmes to 'implement the new proposed curricula' (Akoulouse et al, 2001). In some studies, like Rivers and Aggleton (1999), there is a suggestion that teachers need to be considered as sexual beings who themselves might have difficulty teaching sex education. However, these studies' response regarding what is necessary is reductionist and assumes a linearity about the relationship between knowledge and skills that is devoid of context and culture, on the one hand, and that underplays teachers as active agents, on the other. The following suggestion illustrates this:

> Policies and programmes are needed to transfer skills teachers need in order for them to feel confident to teach about HIV/AIDS and issues of sexuality. This implies that teacher training address the specific needs and circumstances of teachers in the workplace. We emphasize that HIV/AIDS is a workplace issue for teachers and there is a need for a comprehensive support system that would enable teachers to perform their duties and yet deal with their own personal situation (Akoulouze et al, 2001:23).

Few studies take account of teachers' lives as a key mediating factor in the teaching (delivery) of HIV/AIDS. It would seem that an assumption is made that if they (teachers) have the necessary knowledge and skills to teach, they *will*, *can* and *will want to* teach effectively, notwithstanding how they position themselves (or are positioned) within the HIV/AIDS discourse. Neglected, too, is how these teachers are positioned in and out of school and how within such spaces, cultural and social practices shape their experience and understanding of the disease. More importantly, within the current research agenda, there is a lack of an interrogation of teachers as active agents working (shaping and being shaped) within contested and contestable discourses where they can — and, indeed do — make choices about what knowledge to teach, when and how. Therefore, where teachers have been the focus of study, it has been teachers as objects of a structure and system (deliverers of curricula) that has been the issue, rather than teachers as individuals who work and live in contexts in and to which they themselves are contributors, shapers, negotiators and mediators.

Context and culture and HIV/AIDS

Sontag (1990) has suggested that the ways in which we understand HIV/AIDS are more indicative of our broader societal discourse of politics and economy than of any salient features of the disease itself. The discourses of tradition and modernity may seem to play an important role here, where alternatively modernity in terms of women's behaviour and tradition in terms of male sexuality are played out as the culprits behind the prevalence of the disease. When HIV/AIDS is blamed on the 'modern' behaviour of women and when control is reasserted over women's bodies in virginity testing through the contemporary reinvention of traditional practice, this becomes an expression of an anxiety over the relationship between tradition and modernity. The rediscovery of a certain cultural stereotype of black South Africans, and of African culture in general, can be related to early colonial and apartheid definitions of the 'other' (Steinberg et al, 2002). On the other hand, while cultural essentialism should be discarded, the interventions in school are almost completely devoid of any acknowledgement of cultural and contextual aspects that clearly play an important, and sometimes a detrimental, role in negotiations and decision making with regard to sex. What seems obvious is that there is an urgent need to examine deeply held beliefs and practices about sex and everyday sexual practices in such a way that this cultural knowledge can be used in a meaningful way in terms of interventions in the field of education. Moreover, the relationship between sex and the socioeconomic situation needs closer examination. The complex relationship between knowledge and behaviour is acknowledged as being a problem, and it would seem necessary therefore for research to be located within situated contexts in which the youth and teachers construct their sexual identities and make sense of HIV/AIDS-related messages, rather than only finding out what they know about the disease.

Conclusion

From this review, it seems clear that three key elements are left unaccounted for in the research on HIV/AIDS and education. The first is the lack of a critical engagement with the concept of culture and how, through this silence, culture is either misinterpreted as fixed and static, essentialised or conflated with ethnicity and language. The second element highlights how, in the research agenda issue of context, culture and the core of the problem — ie what happens at the chalk face in schools — have been left largely unattended. Our suspicion is that the failure of many of HIV/AIDS educational programmes is at least partly due to the lack of culturally appropriate content and approaches, but also because developers of programmes dare to question various detrimental cultural and social practices. The final aspect relates to the methodological framework within which educational research on HIV/AIDS has been framed. Fundamentally, the epistemological questions posed within this sector remain driven by medical, economic and political discourses. These, as we have argued, are primarily shaped by a need to know the *what* rather than to understand the deeply discursive situated contexts where people come to know. In asking different sets of questions, researchers might develop deeper understandings of why, in the midst of readily available information about HIV/AIDS, youth still find themselves unable to negotiate safe sex practices and why teachers are still challenged in teaching about HIV/AIDS.

Chapter 2

Jean Baxen
University of Cape Town

What Questions? HIV/AIDS Educational Research: Beyond More of the Same to Asking Different Epistemological Questions[1]

Introduction

The prevalence of HIV/AIDS among heterosexual populations in sub-Saharan Africa is one of the highest in the world. As one of the countries in sub-Saharan Africa, South Africa has not been left unscathed. As a consequence, with more than 4.5 million of its population already infected, this country faces serious economic, political and social challenges.

A report by the World Health Organisation estimates that 50% of all new HIV infections are among young people, with 30% of the 40 million HIV-infected people being youth in the age group 15–24 years. Estimates are that at least 7 000 young people are infected daily (Gacoin, 2006). Of concern is that many are unaware of their status or that of their sexual partners. This scenario plays itself out along similar lines among youth in sub-Saharan Africa, who are among the fastest growing HIV-infected population. In this region, they make up at least 80% of those currently living with HIV/AIDS (Gallant & Maticka-Tyndale, 2003). This segment of the population in South Africa is also the hardest hit, with researchers suggesting that up to 60% of HIV infections occur within this age group, ie before the age of 25 (Abt Associates, 2001).

As has already been stated in the previous chapter, education, particularly formal education, has long since been recognised and accepted as a key strategy in the fight against HIV/AIDS, not only in South Africa, but around the world (Kelly, 2000; Coombe, 2000; Gallant & Maticka-Tyndale, 2003).

In essence, schools are seen as 'natural' vehicles for knowledge transmission. While this may be true, few questions are posed about two interrelated issues that this chapter addresses. The first relates to assumptions about schools and the second has to do with the epistemological and methodological orientations of research and the type of questions posed in research on HIV/AIDS, particularly in the field of education.

Relating to the schools, few questions are posed about what happens in classrooms. Still fewer questions are raised about *who* mediates knowledge about HIV/AIDS.

[1] A version of this paper appears in *UWC Papers in Education Journal* (Baxen, 2005). The author expresses gratitude for permission to reprint here.

Few studies (eg Baxen, 2006) address the question of how knowledge is produced and what happens to teachers and students in the mediation process. Little is known about how students and teachers are positioned; or, indeed, how they position themselves in the process of mediation when HIV/AIDS is the topic under discussion. This chapter argues that the questions of how and where knowledge is produced seem to be unaccounted for in the development and delivery of messages about HIV/AIDS in schools. Instead, simplistic associations are made about the relationship between mediator and knowledge, with the former presented as a mere deliverer and the latter as uncontested content that is easily communicated to a captive audience.

From a methodological perspective, this chapter examines how educational research on HIV/AIDS follows trends in health and economic settings that have their roots in functionalist epistemologies that, while helpful during the initial phases of the pandemic, fail to account for the material and social conditions within which the pandemic is embedded. As was illustrated in the first chapter of this book, much of the current educational research emphasises *what* people know rather than *how* they come to know, produce and reproduce what they know. This work leaves unattended the importance of the social and cultural contexts in which people make meaning of their lives in relation to the pandemic. Put differently, few if any studies examine the conditions under which teachers and students understand, interpret and experience their actions in relation to HIV/AIDS. Making an epistemological argument, the second part of this chapter argues for an orientation that accounts for the situatedness and contextual embeddedness of the pandemic.

Schools as repositories of interventions and information about HIV/AIDS

For reasons already stated in chapter 1, schools are the most obvious spaces for intervention and prevention programmes, as well as for the delivery of information about HIV/AIDS. In this regard, three elements are evident in a cursory examination of current impact and intervention studies research carried out in sub-Saharan Africa and internationally.

The first is an emphasis on youth either as a 'high-risk group', vulnerable, or sexually active, or, at the very least, sexually aware, and therefore, by implication, a 'natural' target of prevention and intervention programmes (Baxen & Breidlid, 2004). The epistemological questions informing the development of such programmes deal primarily with *what* knowledge youth need in order to make informed decisions about their sexual practices. Responses often lead to programmes providing youth with *more information* and are premised on the assumption that more information will lead to better decision making and well-informed sexual choices. This information, though, is largely biological and emphasises the nature of the virus and how it is contracted and transmitted. It also foregrounds the physical consequences of the disease. Emphasis is usually on 'the body' as flesh, as a physical entity, without desires, feelings and a complex set of circumstances within which it operates.

The limitation of operating within a narrow paradigmatic framework is three-fold. First, and by inference, authority is placed on the 'individual physical body' operating independently within relatively agreeable environments. Second, a reductionist view of the association between knowledge and behaviour is assumed. Third, within such biomedical and interventionist discourses, little attention is given to the social and cultural contexts in which messages are received, produced, reproduced and mediated. This lack of attention to context assigns little significance to the social embeddedness and discursive nature of the disease. As Crewe (2002:450) states regarding the field of sociology, educational research, too, has not sought to 'look critically at how society and the individuals within it are constructed, how they understand power, relationships and education, and how they understand either the epidemic or the attempts to address it'. The emphasis in intervention programmes on the biomedical nature of the disease obscures critical considerations of the pandemic as a social disease that forces players within social contexts to confront both themselves and their sexual identities, behaviours and practices in particular ways.

Emphasis on the 'individual physical body' and the associated silence regarding context also raises other questions about the relationship between agency and structure. Linear associations between knowledge and behaviour, an assumption upon which many of the interventions are premised, obscure the complex and discursive relationship between the individual and the social environment, between the individual and the collective, and between the self and the 'other'. In addressing the paucity of research that goes beyond 'knowledge about HIV/AIDS among youth', LeClerc-Madlala (2002a) expresses the need for new research trends and, by implication, intervention programmes that involve a shift from an emphasis on 'more knowledge' to enabling youth to understand constructions of self and sexual identity in contexts where issues of gender, power and sexuality are connected to constructions of safe sex and negotiation within relationships and HIV/AIDS knowledge. It is in such contexts that, in the face of HIV/AIDS, youth's vulnerability is exacerbated. To address this problematic, and instead of following dominant trends in HIV/AIDS research, it is important that educational research places emphasis not only on the corporeality of the body, but also on the embodiment of specific social and cultural practices in which the body lives and experiences. It is a body with desires; a thinking, feeling, acting body that has the capacity to exercise choice. At the same time, it is one that is sometimes constrained by those very practices. Research therefore has to pay attention to where and how individuals produce themselves, ie the conditions under which they act and respond to information about the pandemic. This means a re-focus on research that understands individuals as operating within complex discursive spaces that often constrain these individuals, while at the same time offering multiple possibilities for making the self.

The second element is associated with the assumption that the majority of youth within the formal schooling sector are located, for the most part, in *secondary* schools, with primary school children often portrayed as asexual and thus not in need of interventions that focus on sexual behaviour (also see chapter 7). The upshot is the neglect of primary schools as a 'key cultural arena for the production of sexuality and sexual identities' (Renold, 2000:309). This, despite research showing that interventions have the most success before sexual debut (Rivers & Aggleton, 1999), on the one hand, and that primary schools are significant sites for the construction and reproduction of sexual identity among children (Mac an Ghail, 1996), on the other. As Baxen and Breidlid (2004:18) suggest:

> the omission of such considerations viewed against the backdrop of where HIV/AIDS prevalence is highest: developing countries, in which many people, especially girls, leave school after

primary school and where the attendance of girl-children is irregular (Rivers & Aggleton, 1999) and in some cases low, brings into sharp focus the limitation of such research foci.

The third element concerns the mediators of knowledge in schools, ie teachers. In the main, there is a paucity of work focusing on them, either as mediators in the intervention process or as a subjects and objects of research. As subjects of research within intervention programmes (eg Akoulouze, Rugalema & Khanye, 2001), teachers have been positioned as deliverers of an uncontested, already negotiated (and agreed upon) body of HIV/AIDS knowledge within schools and institutions that are not presented as discursive, complex and negotiated spaces. In this regard, teachers have then been the targets of training programmes and are portrayed as primarily lacking *knowledge and skills* to teach life skills or other sex education programmes effectively (Baxen & Breidlid, 2004). Other studies (eg Coombe, 2000) attempt to describe teachers as more 'vulnerable' than the rest of society, citing mobility as a key indicator. Others, like Bennel (2003), have repudiated this assumption by providing evidence that makes the argument of teacher vulnerability unsustainable (Baxen & Breidlid, 2004).

Implicitly, assumptions are made that teachers are able, willing and in the 'best' position to mediate knowledge about HIV/AIDS. Explicitly, through clear articulation in the *Revised National Curriculum Statements* (DoE, 2003b) of what knowledge has to be taught at the different levels of general education, teachers are positioned as those who can mediate knowledge about the 'deeply private' in the public arena of the classroom. As we have seen in the section entitled 'Teachers and HIV/AIDS' in chapter 1, few studies consider teachers as individuals, producers, interpreters, reproducers, mediators and purveyors of knowledge and safe sex messages who work within discursive fields where this knowledge is contested and is often considered secret and/or private. In other words, few studies take account of teachers as the embodiment of the gendered, raced, and classed social and cultural practices of the communities in which they live and the schools in which they teach — complex spaces that shape teachers' individual and professional identities. Such omissions thus ignore an important determinant in the success or failure of intervention programmes. For the most part, functionalist orientations position teachers as responsive rather than active agents who are able to make choices in and outside the classroom.

Research questions in educational research on HIV/AIDS

Chapter 1 provided an overview of research on education and HIV/AIDS in Southern Africa in the last decade. While the geographic contexts, target groups and sites have varied in research regarding the first category of studies (KAP studies; see chapter 1), the fundamental research questions are those driven by a need to answer the question: '*What* knowledge, attitudes and practices do different sets of people carry about the pandemic?' Fundamentally, the assertion is that having access to the results of such surveys may lead researchers and programme developers to respond by either providing more knowledge, or, at the very least, developing intervention programmes that bear in mind the knowledge deficits of particular groups. These studies presuppose simplistic links between knowledge and behaviour that do not always yield success in terms of behaviour change.

The second category includes studies that have traced the potential impact of the pandemic on the education sector. The merit of these studies lies in their contribution to awareness raising and responses at the systemic levels of education. From a systemic and institutional perspective, therefore, the general response has been alarm concerning the results, and a response through, for example, establishing HIV/AIDS co-ordinators within national and provincial departments of education.

Representation of disease in educational research on HIV/AIDS

The social representation of HIV/AIDS is rooted in the broader discourses of the 'other' in Third World contexts. Through its (re)presentation as a disease with catastrophic consequences, the research described in chapter 1 inadvertently supports dominant discourses that situate HIV/AIDS as a predominantly African — in fact, *black* African — disease. Thus, like research in sociology, epidemiology, economics and medicine, studies in educational research also seem to be influenced by and embedded in views about Third World contexts and HIV/AIDS as an 'African epidemic' (Crewe, 2002). Crewe (2002:447) states that:

> Discourse about AIDS in the Third World equates the Third World with the savage, the alien or the incomprehensible, and then asserts, by way of contrast, the importance of reason and control (Treichler, 1999:101). These 'Western eyes' from which HIV/AIDS is read, represents Africa and by implications Africans, as irrational and the pandemic as 'incomprehensible, catastrophic and unpredictable'.

This is a view that is supported unintentionally by the studies reviewed in chapter 1.

Methodological frameworks in education research on HIV/AIDS

At this stage of its history, the pandemic affects Third World environments the most, yet Western research frameworks, largely influenced and dominated by religious and medical discourses about disease, drive the research agenda. These discourses, which privilege positivist, scientific, analytical frameworks, constrain the nature of the epistemological questions posed. Often, the primary epistemological questions are those concerned with *what* knowledge can be solicited about the disease, with the emphasis on wanting '*to know*' more about what the information others hold about the disease. The upshot is a proliferation of survey-type research studies that seek to gain an understanding of the knowledge, attitudes and beliefs of particular groups of respondents in various contexts. The limitations of such epistemological frames of references are threefold. At the outset, presuppositions are made about knowledge production and social action. Little attention is paid to the social and cultural contexts in which individuals act and make individual and/or collective identities. The second limitation relates to the dominant discourses of sexuality, religion and medicine that frame the questions posed. By and large, these foreground the biological nature of the disease, with emphasis on its effects on the physical body. Neglect of the social nature of the disease highlights the third important limitation, namely the nexus among sexuality, race, class and HIV/AIDS, and how these are constituted within unequal power relations. As Crewe states (2002:450):

> dealing with AIDS raises all kinds of social, racial and cultural issues that have not been dealt with, such as the sexual behaviour and sexualities of men, the position of women in society,

the sexualities of women, patriarchal behaviour and domestic violence, the sexualities of young people and their perceptions of their future.

While the field of education has only recently entered the field of research in HIV/AIDS, rather than a critique of the dominant epistemological and methodological frameworks of the research to date, this field has merely followed and applied the same dominant frameworks, thus producing more of the same, with similar results and consequences for policy and the development and content of intervention programmes. Crewe (2002:452) corroborates this view by stating that 'the information/belief model', which in my view is *informed* by biomedical and/or religious paradigms, 'operates from the assumption that information about something as serious as AIDS will translate into behaviour change. It argues that rational decision making will come from ensuring access to information'.

Conclusion

This chapter argues for the reorientation of the research agenda to one that questions the nature of research questions, as well as the epistemological and methodological frames of references shaping research in the field of HIV/AIDS in contexts that are different to those where the pandemic first manifested itself. The argument is made that there is a need for a research agenda that goes beyond finding out *what* people know about the pandemic to one that examines *who* these people are and *how* they come to know, act, reproduce and position themselves in relation to this knowledge. Such an orientation begins with different sets of epistemological assumptions and questions that take serious account of the situated and discursive nature of the disease.

Chapter 3

Anders Breidlid
Oslo University College

HIV/AIDS, Cultural Constraints and Educational Intervention Strategies

Introduction

According to the latest Joint UN Action Plan on HIV/AIDS statistics, an estimated 5.5 million South Africans are infected with HIV (UNAIDS, 2006a). The virus is unevenly distributed among the various population groups in South Africa, being most prevalent among the black population, almost six times as frequent as among the second worst affected population group, ie the coloured group. What is even more alarming is the steady increase in the prevalence rate among black people, in a context of decline among other population groups (Chirambo, 2008:144).

Table 3.1: HIV/AIDS prevalence in South Africa (%)

Population	Older than 2 years	15–24 years	15–49 years
Black	13.3	12.3	19.9
White	0.6	0.3	0.5
Coloured	1.9	1.7	3.2
Indian	1.6	0.8	1.0
Male	8.2	4.4	11.7
Female	13.3	16.9	20.2
Total	10.8	10.3	16.2

Source: HSRC (2005)

The seriousness of this situation can be illustrated by projections indicating life expectancy with or without AIDS, figures that will affect black people the most. According to the UN Development Programme and the US Bureau of Census (Chirambo, 2008:147), the life expectancy projections for South Africans without AIDS in 2010 is 68.3 years and with AIDS, 35.5 years. The counter-factuality of these figures notwithstanding, they nevertheless signal a bleak future if interventions fail to make a difference.

Since the prevalence rate is much higher among blacks than other population groups, one aim of this chapter is to discuss some of the challenges in dealing with HIV/AIDS by situating the issue contextually and culturally.

There are a number of conceptual issues that arise from the literature on cultural values, and on cultural values and HIV/AIDS. The most significant is an essentialist orientation in the use of the term 'culture' or 'traditional culture' to signify African culture. In the South African research context, the extent to which differences in the behaviour of adolescents, for example, can be attributable to aspects other than a narrow definition of the terms is not always clear. It would seem that some studies compare the behaviour of adolescents using language or ethnicity as key variables, without considering that these are not always indicative of the practices from which the group is drawn (eg Wood & Jewkes, 1997; Tillotson & Maharaj, 2001). Other studies infer that the results are indicative of a specific culture's values (eg LeClerc Madlala, 2001a; 2002; Breidlid, 2002).

As has been noted in relation to the Xhosa culture:

> There is a sense that despite the intertextuality and dialogic exchange between various value systems, the indigenous cultural values are retained, not only as a means of social cohesion, or as a kind of low-key cultural resistance, but as a fundamental element of Xhosa identity construction (Breidlid, 2002:43).

While it is acknowledged that tradition is often subsumed in modern practices, and vice versa, tension can exist where communities are still very traditional and youth are influenced both by tradition and modernity, thereby making difficult the challenge of navigating their way within social and cultural practices that are fluid and sometimes contradictory (Breidlid, 2002).

This difficulty notwithstanding, this chapter suggests that cultural practices impact seriously on the spread of HIV/AIDS in Southern Africa and that various intervention programmes have been largely ineffective in halting this development, since they have not taken cognisance of cultural factors and since the interventions have often been put across in a culturally insensitive language. Admittedly, changing cultural practices is very difficult, even in the face of this serious pandemic.

A number of South African studies acknowledge explicitly or implicitly the importance of cultural context in the efficacy of intervention programmes. Cohen (2002), for example, suggests that cultural aspects present serious constraints in the attempt to fight the pandemic (besides socioeconomic circumstances), and Archie-Booker, Cervero and Langone (1999) state that HIV/AIDS prevention education must be responsive to culture in order to be effective.

However, not only is the *impact* of cultural beliefs on sexual behaviour, negotiation and change not always clearly spelled out, but the use of cultural knowledge in intervention programmes also seems to be more or less absent. The reason for this may be the sensitive nature of HIV/AIDS as a disease that invokes issues of sex, sexuality and disease that many communities, due to aspects of class, ethnicity and gender, struggle with. In South Africa, a nation striving to achieve a national identity that transcends former differences, such discussions may also be deemed politically incorrect. The seriousness of the pandemic means, however, that such cultural and political considerations must be approached more creatively in an attempt to design more efficient strategies.

Cultural constraints in fighting HIV/AIDS

Cohen's (2002) suggestion that there are serious cultural constraints in fighting the pandemic is an important point of departure for the discussion that follows. The discussion starts by exploring the so-called Caldwell hypothesis that African sexuality is different from Eurasian sexuality. It proceeds to discuss cultural sexual traits in Africa more specifically, with a particular emphasis on Southern Africa and the myths surrounding the prevention of HIV/AIDS infection among certain population groups. Third, the South African government's policies on HIV/AIDS are explored, focusing particularly on the ideological and cultural content of strategies linked to prevention programmes. Finally, the chapter explores the role of education as a site for knowledge transmission and queries to what extent the correlational link between knowledge and behaviour is addressed in educational intervention programmes.

The Caldwell hypothesis

While there is a danger in projecting age-old Western stereotypes and prejudices onto African cultures, there is also the risk of evading the whole topic of African sexuality and simply talking of preventive measures that are often Western in approach and origin.

Caldwell, Caldwell and Quiggin (1989:187) argue that 'there is a distinct and internally coherent African system embracing sexuality, marriage, and much else, and that it is no more right or wrong, progressive or unprogressive than the Western system'. They further argue that there are certain elements of African cultural practices with a bearing on sexual behaviour that may have adverse consequences in the age of HIV/AIDS. According to these researchers, aspects of sexual behaviour are not placed at the centre of African moral, religious and social systems, nor do such systems sanctify chastity (Caldwell et al, 1989:194), in deep contrast to the focus on sexual behaviour and chastity and the tremendous solemnity regarding sex in large segments of the Euro-North American population. The impression is that attitudes towards the sexual act are simple and straightforward, and that virtue is related more to 'success in reproduction than to limiting profligacy' (Caldwell et al, 1989:188), with reproduction being a central element in indigenous African religion. The touchstone of the contrast between Eurasia and Africa is not male but female sexuality. Caldwell et al (1989:197) state that:

> A pragmatic attitude exists in Africa toward the latter, with a fair degree of permissiveness toward premarital relations that are not blatantly public, and a degree of acceptance that surreptitious extramarital relations are not the high point of sin and usually should not be severely punished.

There is no indication that either female premarital chastity or male sexual abstention has been supported by religious sanctions. Moreover, the claim is that many African societies admire risk taking, especially dashing behaviour by young men (Caldwell et al, 1989:224–25).

Sickness and death are most often not considered natural events, but ascribed to evil spirits and breaches of taboos, and are, therefore, explained not in the behaviour that led to them, but in relation to who or what caused the sick person's misfortune. When the risk of contracting HIV/AIDS is recognised within this framework of understanding, Caldwell (1999:11) finds that

> even many who recognise the role of infection and pathogens believe they are merely the intermediary mechanisms .... In these circumstances there is little point in avoiding the one type of infection only to find that the malevolent forces settle for another mechanism.

The situation is aggravated by the commonly held belief that one's time to die was decided long ago, or that one will die in the not too distant future anyway. 'Some men practicing high-risk sex say that, if the latency period is a decade, they are not worried because they are likely to die of something else in such a long time' (Caldwell, 1999:10–11).

By linking this lack of cautiousness about one's health to what she terms 'non-HIV life expectancy', Oster (2007) finds that responsiveness to risk awareness corresponds to the length of life expectancy without HIV/AIDS. The assumption is somewhat problematic, however, given the huge gap in life expectancy with and without AIDS.

Caldwell's thesis of African sexuality has been contested, most notably by Ahlberg (1994), who claims that Caldwell et al (1989) have left out all data suggesting that 'there was moral restraint attached to sexuality in Africa' (Ahlberg, 1994:223). Ahlberg, by referring to the Kikuyu culture, shows how taboos and regulations 'were extensively used in the maintenance of good conduct' in terms of sexual discipline (Ahlberg, 1994:230). Other African communities had similar regulations (Krige, 1968; Evans-Pritchard, 1965). As Epstein (2007:146) states:

> Just as anywhere else, sexual behaviour on the (African) continent is governed by strict moral rules. They may not be the same as Western rules — polygamy and other forms of long-term concurrency are considered acceptable to many people — but they are rules all the same.

This is in line with Mbiti (1969), who also claims that there was no anarchy in terms of sexual norms. Sexual offences were taken very seriously: 'when adultery is dealt with it is seriously dealt with .... Fornication, incest, rape, seduction, homosexual relations, sleeping with a forbidden "relative" or domestic animals, intimacy between relatives ... all constitute sexual offences in a given community' (Mbiti, 1969:147–48).

Sexual culture in Southern Africa

While traditional sexual mores in many communities were highly regulated, Ahlberg claims that during colonialism, 'sexuality was dramatically transformed, from a context where it was open but kept within well defined social control and regulating mechanisms, to being an individual, private matter surrounded largely by silence' (Ahlberg, 1994:233). This led to the existence of two distinct moral systems, 'neither of which has much authority over sexual behaviour' (Ahlberg, 1994:233). Accordingly, there are no simple mechanisms to discipline deviant sexual behaviour or to enforce traditional sexual norms.

While knowledge of traditional sexual regulations is important, particularly in designing alternative intervention strategies, the contemporary sexual practices discussed below are extremely problematic in combating the HIV/AIDS pandemic, whatever the underlying causes for such practices are.

Nattrass (2004:279) acknowledges that sexual culture in Southern Africa is an important dimension relating to the AIDS pandemic. According to her, 'gender inequality, sexual violence, a preference for dry sex, fatalistic attitudes and pressures to prove fertility contribute to a high-risk environment' (Nattrass, 2004:26–27). LeClerc-Madlala is more specific in her discussion of cultural sexual practices by referring to the Zulu sexual culture, which is 'underpinned by meanings which associate sex with gifts and manliness with the ability to attract and maintain multiple sex partners' (LeClerc-Madlala, 2002:31–32). This clearly contributes to the spread of HIV. LeClerc-Madlala (2001a:41) goes on to characterise the Zulu culture in terms of

> gender inequity, transactional sex, the socio-cultural *isoka* of multiple sexual partners, lack of discussion of both men and women to accept sexual violence as 'normal' sexual behaviour along with the 'right' of men to control sexual encounters, and the existence of increasingly discordant and contested gender scripts.

Other problematic cultural traits refer to the practice where young women form sexual liaisons with older men for financial advantage and where sex is a currency with which African women and girls are frequently expected to pay in a desperate situation. 'Many believe that there is no romance without finance'.

Nattrass refers to Zambia, where women, educated about the virus, nevertheless offered sex during a famine because they would rather die of AIDS than of hunger (*Mail & Guardian,* 1–7 November 2002, in Nattrass, 2004:27). This means that they may be more exposed to contracting diseases, thus making them vulnerable to HIV infection. This is particularly so in relationships based on exchange or money, because it is under such circumstances where young women have little power to insist on condom usage (Kelly & Ntlabati, 2002:52).

Added to these cultural sexual practices are the myths surrounding the disease and the possible cures put forward. While some myths are harmless ('African potato cures AIDS'), others are critically dangerous to the spreading of HIV, particularly the myth that having sex with a virgin or a baby will provide a cure. Moreover, misconceptions that HIV can be caused by witchcraft weaken intervention strategies, as well as the current debate about whether forced sex is rape or simply sex (Mandela, 2002:82).[1] These myths and misconceptions have sprung out of cultural beliefs that are nurtured by an indigenous epistemology based on magic and supernatural phenomena and explanations. Such myths are associated with the reported increase in child rape and the sharp increase of HIV among young girls. The strength and pervasiveness of this myth is, however, disputed (Nattrass, 2004:141).

Poverty poses another challenge to combating the pandemic. According to the UN Development Programme, South Africa is becoming increasingly unequal, and 'more people were living in poverty in 2002 than 1995' (Chirambo, 2008:147). Statistics show that provinces with higher levels of poverty also have higher levels of HIV/AIDS, and this correlation shows the 'relevance of including poverty as a contextual variable in any social science discussion of the epidemic' (Chirambo, 2008:147). To the extent that women's sexual behaviour is a product of economic circumstances, interventions at the level of individual behaviour and sexual culture are unlikely to be very successful.

1 These beliefs seem to be fairly pervasive within certain ethnic groups where forced sex is not seen as coercion. The longer the relationship, the more 'right' a male has to demand sex from the 'submissive' female. Should she resist, he has the cultural 'right' to beat her into submission. Cultural systems carry immense gender inequalities.

The link between poverty and sexual behaviour poses another major challenge for AIDS interventions.

Sexual culture and ethnicity

The cultural sexual practices referred to above are often associated with black African culture, and are, if Caldwell et al (1989) are anything to go by, different from Euroasian sexuality. Nattrass (2004) questions this difference by referring to a qualitative study by Marcus (2000). Marcus found that it was usual among white university students in South Africa to engage in multiple partnering (both serial and concurrent), as well as casual sex for its own sake (Marcus 2000:32; see chapter 9 in this book). Marcus' research notwithstanding, there seems to be no study on white sexual behaviour in South Africa that makes the link between cultural sexual practices and the spread of HIV. Literature does not regularly link myths and magic with HIV/AIDS prevalence when white populations are the target.

Pointedly, a district survey in the Western Cape province (*Mail & Guardian Online*, 13 October 2004, in Nattrass, 2004:27) carried out at 374 facilities and involving the testing of 5 964 people revealed that the black townships of Gugulethu and Nyanga had a prevalence rate of HIV of 28.1% and Khayelitsha 27.2%, far above other districts in the Western Cape. While the prevalence of HIV follows ethnic lines, it is worth noting that it also seems to follow income groups and education levels. Both Gugulethu, Nyanga and Khayelistsha are townships with relatively low income and education levels, thus upholding the view of a correlation between poverty and the escalation in HIV rates. While African households in the Western Cape have an average annual household income of R33 449, white households averaged R165 320 (Provincial Decision-making Enabling Project, 2005). According to Nattrass, and since malnutrition and parasitic infection increase HIV susceptibility, there is a good reason for assuming that poverty is a breeding ground for the spread of HIV in sub-Saharan Africa (Nattrass, 2004:29).

Levels of education are also noted to be an indicator of HIV infection. A national survey of South African youth reported that there were lower reported levels of sexual activity among better educated youth. Those with tertiary educational qualifications had lower rates, and 'those in high skill bands have relatively low levels of HIV infection' (Nattrass, 2004:30).

Government policies

Inadequate responses by most African governments have no doubt contributed, and are still contributing to the AIDS pandemic. The often conflicting messages by the Presidency in South Africa has resulted in messages about infection not being taken seriously, thus weakening the impact of intervention programmes. The defensive re-action by the government to criticism of its HIV/AIDS policies limits the possibility of engaging with and improving on government's capacity to implementing the policies. It has been detrimental to government policies in that opportunities were missed to obtain evaluative input that may have led to improvement in and better implementation of the nation's HIV/AIDS policies.

This notwithstanding, the South African government's policies regarding the pandemic are changing at a slow, but steady pace. In its *The HIV/AIDS Emergency: Guidelines for Educators* (DoE, 2000/02), it is acknowledged that the HIV pandemic is an emergency that would have serious consequences for the education sector:

> If the current rate of infection does not slow down, by the year 2010 one in every four people in the country will have HIV. In ten years, the disease will have made orphans of three-quarters of a million South African children.

The *Guidelines* (DoE, 2000/02) also acknowledges that the disease is spreading so fast 'mainly because many South Africans, especially men, are careless about their sexual behaviour .... This means that the death rate from HIV/AIDS is still climbing rapidly among men and women of all ages, especially among sexually-active people'. The document warns that 'unless we take the necessary precautions any one of us may contract HIV'. The *Guidelines* concur with statements by other researchers early on that acknowledge the role of social and economic circumstances in the increase of HIV prevalence.

The *Guidelines* (DoE, 2000/02) also focus on the role of culture and ways in which some cultural practices may be detrimental to HIV prevention. This policy document raises concerns about how some cultural practices are being taken up and the consequences this has for responses to combating the spread of the pandemic:

> HIV/AIDS is a new disease that was not there when our old customs were created. The arrival of HIV means we have to make some changes to our culture because if we do not make these changes very large numbers of our young people may die and we may do so as well. Changing the rules about discussing sex does not mean that our culture will be threatened. There is much more to our culture than codes and practices relating to sex. In fact, cultures change all the time. That is how it survives .... We need to adapt our customary attitude toward sex and talking about sex, because the lives of our spouses and partners, our children, and those in our care, depend upon us (DoE, 2000/02).

The message in this document also refers to aspects of religious beliefs that are detrimental in relation to the present HIV pandemic: 'Some of our religious beliefs about sexual morality may make it difficult for us to discuss sex with children, but we cannot expose young people in our care to life-threatening situations when we have information that could save them.' Moreover, the message stresses the moral aspects involved: 'The threat of HIV does not mean to discard our moral code. A strong and clear moral code was never more necessary' (DoE, 2000/02). This emphasis on the moral aspects is important in a situation where the government's HIV campaigns have been criticised for being too technical and too modern in their approach.

Strategies to combat the pandemic are varied. To what extent do these strategies take into account how cultural practices not only affect responses to intervention programmes, but also how the implicit and explicit messages they attempt to convey are received?

The *HIV/AIDS/STD Strategic Plan for South Africa 2000–2005* (South Africa, 2000:16) calls for 'an effective and culturally appropriate information, education and communications (IEC) strategy'. This notwithstanding, the implementation of the plan seems, to a large extent, focused either on the use of condoms or on improving access to and the use of male and female condoms, especially among 15–25 year olds (South Africa, 2000:19).

The ABC strategy that prioritises 'A' for abstinence, 'B' for be faithful and 'C' for use of condoms has been criticised in some quarters in South Africa for paying too little attention to abstinence and faithfulness and placing too much reliance on condoms, especially as regards the allocation of resources in terms of funds spent on their purchase, distribution and promotion.

The reason for the focus on condom distribution is not necessarily due to a sexual liberation ideology, but more likely due to the acknowledgement that changes in sexual behaviour take a long time and are very difficult, and that 'safe' sex is an urgent priority, even if deeply rooted sexual practices (other than condom use) are not changed. Questions about the cultural appropriateness of such an approach are often not in question, particularly when a common response among youth is that 'using a condom is the same as eating a banana with the peel on.'

The new *HIV/AIDS and Sexually Transmitted Infection (STI) Strategic Plan for South Africa (NSP 2007–2011)* (DoH, 2007) expands on the above and emphasises the gender problematic and human rights protection. It is a comprehensive plan intended to address the multiple challenges across a wide range of sectors, including areas of prevention, treatment, care and support; human and legal rights; and monitoring, research and surveillance (Chirambo, 2008:142).

Awareness programmes and cultural appropriateness

The cultural appropriateness of the probably most commonly known awareness campaign in South Africa, loveLife,[2] has also been hotly debated. Planned Parenthood and the Planned Parenthood Association of South Africa (PPASA)[3] are providers, with the former positioning itself as a sexual health provider and educator. They offer sexual health services from abortions, contraception and sex education curricula to lobbying governments to legalise abortion. LoveLife is primarily focused on mass media campaigning and has a budget of over R600 million annually, mainly accessed from the Bill and Melinda Gates Foundation; the Kaiser Foundation; the South African government; the UN Children's Fund; the Nelson Mandela Foundation; and the Global Fund on HIV/AIDS, TB and Malaria. However, it claims to be more than a mass media campaign. Apart from the regular adverts and inserts it places on billboards and in national newspapers (such as 'Thetha-Nathi' and 'S'camtoPRINT' in *The Sunday Times*), it also makes use of television and radio to raise awareness.

LoveLife has an 'in your face' approach to HIV/AIDS and sexuality. Its vision is to 'reduce the rate of HIV infection among 15–20 year olds by 50% in five years'. This will be achieved by combining high-powered media awareness and education with adolescent-friendly reproductive health services. The entire strategy is premised on the notion that if people talk openly about sex, they will practise safer sex. LoveLife believes that it is impossible to change behaviour, but it is possible to change attitudes.

A fundamental awareness raising strategy by LoveLife has been the use of billboard messaging. However, this strategy has not been without controversy. While initial per-

2 LoveLife is a branch of the 'mother organisation'.
3 PPASA is referred to within most loveLife publications with the phrase, 'loveLife's initiatives are implemented by a consortium of leading non-governmental organisations'. PPASA is one of these NGOs.

mission to run advertisements was not given as a result of the advertisements being perceived as offensive, culturally inappropriate, and encouraging promiscuity and early sexual activity, the government rescinded its objections on the grounds that the messaging was intended to encourage discussion among the target audience — the youth.

However, loveLife's own surveys have revealed that as few as 27.2% of respondents answered 'yes' to the question of whether the billboards 'caused them to think'. As cursory examination of the reasons why the messages do not have the desired effect may have to do with their lack of specificity and cultural inappropriateness. This may be supported by the response be an AIDS activist organisation, the National Association of People Living with HIV/AIDS (Napwa), which celebrated new year 2003 by vandalising and scrawling 'Napwa' across three loveLife billboards in Germiston. Napwa claimed that 'a lot of money has been pumped into loveLife and they are wasting it on meaningless messages' and that 'the message displayed on their billboards is public pornography and isn't interpreted properly for its target market to understand' (*Mail & Guardian*, 2003).

In a critical article in the *Mail & Guardian*, Leclerc-Madlala points out that South Africa, more than any other African country, has had the benefit of resources to put together a sophisticated media blitz against AIDS, yet the country still has the highest rate of AIDS infections of any country on the African continent. She then points out that the chic images used to reach the youth are those that portray youth 'spiked of hair and pierced of navel, beautiful, hip, straight-talking teens' who, she argues, are more typical of Los Angeles or Glasgow than those more familiar to youth in the local context of urban and rural South Africa. This global approach, she argues, fails to appeal to this complex diversity within the South African context. Rather, it appeals to a 'narrow band of privileged youth' — the 'middle class' — who enjoy 'multi-racial camaraderie in suburban rave clubs' (LeClerc-Madlala, 2002b).

The controversy about loveLife is interesting, since it highlights the cultural complexity of transmitting messages on HIV to a population that is culturally heterogeneous and whose experiences are often shaped, on the one hand by a complex interlinkage between modern and tradition, an intricate intersection of class, gender, race and ethnicity on the other hand. The consequence is often a production of multiple and often conflicting social realities. LoveLife's marketing is modernist and seems at odds with ways of approaching a culturally diverse South African population where the traditional is often subsumed in modernity, as opposed to coexisting outside of a modern space.

HIV/AIDS and education

According to a 2005 survey by the Human Sciences Research Council, 12.7% of teachers in South Africa are HIV-positive. This corresponds to the national statistics, and is confirmed by very high teacher absenteeism (Chirambo, 2008). The regional variance of teacher absenteeism also correlates with the different prevalences in the various provinces, ie teachers from KwaZulu-Natal and Mpumalanga have the highest prevalence rate in the country.

In *The HIV/AIDS Emergency: Guidelines for Educators* (DoE, 2000/02), educators are given a special responsibility along the lines of an ethical model: 'Educators must set an example of responsible sexual behaviour. In so doing, they will protect their families, colleagues, learners and themselves.' The role of the teacher is not, however, without its challenge. Few, if any, studies have been done on the role of teachers in HIV prevention programmes. Are teachers willing and able to teach? Can they teach about sex, sexuality and disease in the public space of the classroom without fear of repercussions from school authorities and communities? What is their positionality regarding this issue? What is their moral position on teaching HIV/AIDS education? These questions are not explored in AIDS education literature and thus assume an easy fit between teachers and the curriculum that is unsustainable.

According to a national review in South Africa of more than 10 000 women under 50 years, a third of rapes of girls are committed by teachers (Jewkes et al, 2002), thus putting doubts on their capacity to not only teach about sex education to children, but also to fill their position of authority as role models. If teachers are sexually abusing children, this is made all the more drastic in that 'South Africa's 443 000 educators constitute the largest occupational group in the country. Since at least 12% are reported to be HIV positive' (Coombe, 2000b:17), it means that over 40 000 teachers are HIV-positive. To give support to these fears, Hickey (2002:599) states:

> Schools, particularly in rural areas, can be a breeding ground for the disease by providing opportunities primarily via sexual relationships between male teachers and young girls. Reportedly the measured infection rate amongst young women between age 15 and 19 rose from 12.7% in 1997 to 21% in 1998.

The DoE (1999:14) states that 'educators may not have sexual relations with learners or students', suggesting a political will to confront teachers who abuse their position and those entrusted to their care. Questions do remain about the consequences for such offences and whether or not punishment is always meted out.

Intervention strategies

In chapter 1, Baxen and Breidlid state that some studies (eg Wood, Maepa & Jewkes, 1997; Levine & Ross, 2002) have sought to examine and gain some understanding of *what* knowledge, attitudes and practices (KAP studies) those participating in the educational endeavour (teachers, youth and adolescents) carry. Often, these studies have as their main outcome recommendations regarding the development of 'effective' prevention strategies for those perceived as 'most vulnerable', which in many instances are youth aged between 14 and 24.

As was stated in chapter 1, there is very little co-ordinated information on what South African youth know about reproductive health. Judging from some of the studies, some South African youth have a *very* sketchy understanding of reproduction, puberty and sexually transmitted diseases (Wood et al, 1997). However, Kelly (2000), in a study commissioned by the Department of Health, found that youth had good access to accurate HIV/AIDS information and were regularly exposed to such information.

Even though Kelly's research might be true in some instances, the educational intervention programmes have not, it seems, been able to effect a positive correlation between knowledge and behaviour. It seems, therefore, that some South Africans are constructing their sexual identity and ideas about safety from infection in a complex, discursive space where competing knowledge systems coexist to produce and reproduce conflicting messages about risk, contraction and infection.

In an attempt to examine ways of increasing the possibility of behavioural change, Wight (1999) found in his study that learner-driven classes do not work as well as teacher-driven ones. Wight argues that there are severe limits to the efficacy of pupil empowerment in sex and HIV/AIDS education. Skinner (2001), however, finds that educators were seen as out of touch with youth. He describes this as another factor distancing youth from scientific information and making them inclined to look to alternative sources of knowledge.

Although a number of studies describe South African cultural beliefs that have a bearing on sexual behaviour, it has been noted that few studies investigate the intersection between either cultural context or cultural beliefs and intervention programme efficacy.

The emphasis on intervention and prevention programmes (giving youth *more* knowledge) referred to above seems to be underpinned by reductionist views of the link between knowledge and behaviour. This view creates a dissociation of the interface between sexual identity, education and HIV/AIDS. More importantly, what it leaves unattended is the deeply complex nature of the social, contextual and cultural discursive fields in which youth receive and interpret the HIV/AIDS messages and how they understand, experience and use this knowledge in the face of or while constructing, performing and playing out their sexual identities.

Louw (1991) argues that the medical model that favours information on safe sexual practices, especially condom use, has achieved some results, but 'it has been shown that information and education campaigns (as in the case of tuberculosis) do not stop the spread of a disease; medical information is not enough in the long run' (Louw, 1991:101). He favours an ethical model as a long-term strategy that might have the desired effects of reducing infection among youth. Such a response does, of course, raise questions about whose ethics and what ethical framework might be applied in a complex context like South Africa. Questions may be posed, therefore, about productions and interpretations of morality and its inclusion in prevention programmes in a context where its constructions are often open to transformation.

The interface of tradition and modernity has had a detrimental impact on some cultural practices. This has resulted in an underplaying of the traditional social support systems in terms of sexual norms and behaviour; aspects that, in some communities, remain intact. Ahlberg's (1994) reference to positive sexual norms and practices in traditional African communities noted earlier is important knowledge in strategic discussions of the pandemic. Therefore, undercommunication of these in discussions of intervention strategies to combat the pandemic can be seen as a factor contributing to HIV/AIDS intervention inefficiency.

Conclusion

Cultural practices are not static. Sontag (1990) suggests that the ways in which we understand HIV/AIDS are, therefore, more indicative of our broader societal discourse of politics and economy than of any salient features of the disease itself. Sexual practices alone cannot explain the virulence of the spread of AIDS in Africa. The combination of cultural, socioeconomic and biomedical factors, together with unsafe sexual practices, produce fertile ground for the spread of HIV.

Prevention programmes thus cannot be limited to certain sectors of society, ie education or health, but must address the multiplicity of areas that critically impact on the spread of HIV and AIDS. Moreover, these interventions must transcend a mere economic and technical discourse and take into account the deeply ingrained cultural factors and practices among the various groups in a complex South African society. While cultural essentialism should be discarded, interventions must acknowledge and identify cultural and contextual aspects that, it has been noted, clearly play an important, and sometimes detrimental, role in the negotiations and decision making with regard to sex.

Further, it would be important to examine the interface between discourses of tradition and modernity in the development of more appropriate intervention strategies that could lead to behaviour change. Such a space would encourage discussions about, for example, how modern concepts of women's behaviour are juxtaposed with traditional conceptions of male sexuality. When HIV/AIDS is blamed, for example, on the 'modern' behaviour of women, and when control is reasserted over women's bodies in virginity testing through the contemporary reinvention of traditional practice, this is the expression of an anxiety over the relationship between tradition and modernity.

The failure of modernist interventions to achieve behavioural change makes it urgent to explore the extent to which traditional processes, practices, dynamics, structures and networks within communities are under-reported and under-utilised as resources to support or facilitate behavioural change. There is a sense that reference to traditional norms and values stands a better chance of being accepted and adhered to than alien, modernist interventions that so far have been met with massive, if tacit, resistance on the behavioural level. Interventions devoid of any acknowledgement of cultural and contextual specificity may be those that would have detrimental consequences for success in reducing the effects of the pandemic.

PART 2

SCHOOLS, COMMUNITY, CULTURE AND CONTEXT

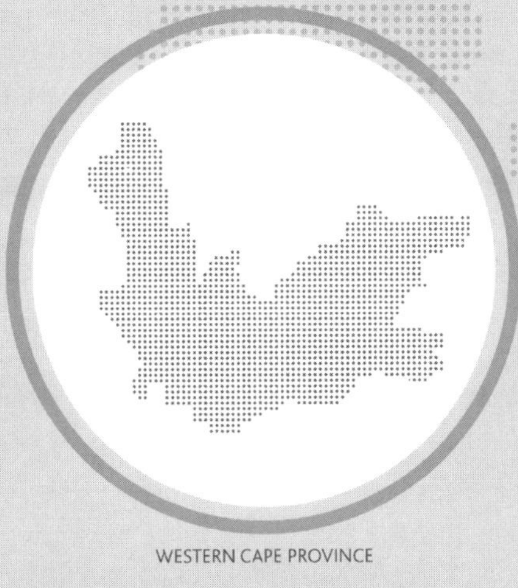

WESTERN CAPE PROVINCE

Chapter 4

Bernice Adonis with Jean Baxen
University of Cape Town

School Culture, Teacher Identity and HIV/AIDS

Introduction

This chapter discusses ways in which the cultures of schools and teachers' personal identities act as filters to the knowledge taught about HIV/AIDS and the process by which children come to know and understand HIV/AIDS messages. More specifically, the chapter focuses on how school cultures and personal histories enable or restrain teachers in their approach to teaching about sexuality and HIV/AIDS. It discusses how teachers, as the embodiment of community social and cultural practices, act from particular positions. For the most part such positioning, we argue, in which individuals are always aware of their membership in a particular culture in and out of school, shapes teachers' professional behaviour, even though it does so differently and for different reasons.

We argue that current educational debates regarding HIV/AIDS focus mostly either on the impact of the pandemic on the education sector at a systemic level (Coombe & Kelly, 2001), pedagogical practices (Mirembe, 2002) or the success of HIV/AIDS education intervention programmes among the youth (Agrawal et al, 1999). Few studies, if any, focus on the context of schooling as a site for the transmission and reproduction of particular forms of HIV/AIDS knowledge. Fewer still focus on school culture and teacher identity as filters through which teachers not only create a professional identity, but also make pedagogical decisions about what and how to teach in lessons on HIV/AIDS and sexuality. Little is known about how, within these institutions, this process is mediated, reproduced, and interpreted. This chapter is based on a study that was conducted in some primary schools in the Western Cape Province, South Africa.

Background and context

In dealing with the HIV/AIDS pandemic, the South African government has had to consider its responses at various levels: politically, socially and educationally. Politically, the stance of the government has been problematic. In its decisions about how to treat and manage the disease, it has often perpetuated confusion and controversy through conflicting and contradictory messages from high-ranking officials. Fuelling this uncertainty have been the public questions raised by President Thabo Mbeki as to whether HIV actually causes AIDS. These questions have entrenched misunderstandings about the identification, causes of and ways of treating HIV/AIDS.

Medically, the response has been more positive, with the development of an integrated healthcare programme that includes treatment, research and care (SouthAfrica.info,

2007). The response from the Department of Social Welfare has included the establishment of social welfare grants for those infected and affected by the disease.

The government has identified education as one of the key strategies to combat the disease. In this regard, the government has embarked on an education drive through its life-skills and HIV/AIDS education programmes, which include a curriculum development process and a mass media drive[1] that endeavours to promote public awareness and healthy sexual behaviour (SouthAfrica.info, 2007). Collaborations between schools and their respective communities have also been encouraged. The idea is that collaborations among schools and parents, care givers, communities and faith-based organisations would facilitate better implementation of HIV/AIDS programmes.

Schools are seen as having a key role to play in informing children about the disease. Schenker and Nyirenda (2002) and Gallant and Maticka-Tyndale (2003) argue that schools are suitable spaces for HIV knowledge dissemination, since they accommodate children between the ages of approximately 5–18 years (with the top end of this range being the ages of high risk of infection).

In recognising the critical role schools can play in disseminating HIV/AIDS knowledge, the Western Cape Education Department (WCED) promulgated several school-focused HIV/AIDS knowledge dissemination and prevention strategies. These strategies include a provincial education policy for HIV/AIDS based on the national policy. For instance, all schools in the Western Cape are required to teach HIV/AIDS and sexuality and provide life-skills education for at least half an hour a week (WCED, 2002). In addition, materials for the teaching of HIV/AIDS are supplied to schools free of charge. The province has also developed a rigorous teacher-training programme for life-skills teachers.

These strategies of the WCED are commendable and, indeed, seem workable. However, what they fail to address is the problematisation of two interrelated issues this chapter addresses, namely, teachers as producers and reproducers of HIV/AIDS knowledge, and schools as sites of delivery of contestable HIV/AIDS messages. Assumptions seem to have been made that (a) teachers merely deliver an already agreed upon body of knowledge and that their own influences and experiences do not act as mediatory tools for what and how they teach; and (b) schools are neutral sites, when, in fact, there is a large body of literature (eg Prosser, 1999; Wyner, 1991) that show schools as deeply ideological places where knowledge is not merely delivered, but contested, produced and reproduced in complex ways.

Methodology

Since this study aimed at gaining a textured understanding of how school culture and personal histories acts as a filter to what knowledge is taught about HIV/AIDS and the process by which children come to know and understand HIV/AIDS messages, it was necessary to locate it within a qualitative paradigm. Two approaches within the qualitative paradigm were employed, namely a combination of phenomenology and narrative. The use of narratives enabled making sense of lived experiences (De la Rey,

[1] Examples include loveLife, Yizo Yizo, supplements in newspapers, and advertisements on radio and television.

1999), while the phenomenological approach was utilised to gain a deep understanding of school culture as a social phenomenon.

This investigation was conducted at three primary schools situated in the Cape Flats area in the Western Cape. It was part of a larger research project on HIV/AIDS and education discussed in the introduction to this book. The three schools were selected from the five primary schools used in the larger study, and were purposively chosen to ensure representation of the diversity of the South African population. They were therefore selected from historically white, coloured/Indian and black areas.

Data were collected using three methods, ie observations, interviews and document analysis. The observations, which lasted three to four weeks per school, involved observing the daily occurrences at the schools; meetings; and interactions among teachers, learners, and teachers and learners. Classroom and lesson observations involving two life-skills teachers in each of the schools were also conducted. Only life-skills lessons were observed, since it was in this learning area that HIV/AIDS mediation mainly took place.

A series of interviews were conducted with life-skills teachers in each school. Minutes of meetings, the school vision and mission statements, curriculum circulars, codes of conduct for staff and learners, and disciplinary procedures are among the documents that were reviewed.

For purposes of confidentiality, all the schools and teachers are referred to by pseudonyms.

Conceptions of culture and school culture

Since the central focus of this chapter is the influence of school culture on teachers' understanding of and pedagogical practices regarding HIV/AIDS, this section explores the concept of culture — particularly notions of school culture and the debates around it.

The term 'culture' conjures up different ideas and meanings. The brief clarification of the term here serves to illuminate what is meant by it when used in relation to the school. As early as 1871, Taylor (in Cashmore, 2004) defined the term 'culture' as 'that complex whole which includes knowledge, beliefs, art, morals, law, custom and any other capabilities and habits acquired by man as a member of society'. According to Bourdieu and Passeron (1977), culture includes beliefs, traditions, values and language. Hofstede (1984) understands culture as a collective (mental) programming of the mind that distinguishes groups of people from one another. To Wyner (1991), culture consists of many small chunks of knowledge that are stored as a large pool of information within a bounded social group. Damen (1987) defines culture as the learned and shared human patterns or models for living, pervading all aspects of human social interactions. These definitions illustrate the variety of opinions about and, by implication, the complexity of the term 'culture'. What is clear, though, is that it is not a single 'thing', but is constituted by countless factors.

Differing schools of thought exist in relation to the notion of school culture. Prosser (1999) conceives school culture as the 'overall' character of a school. He postulates that each school has a 'different reality or mindset of school life' (Prosser, 1999:3). Dalin, Rolff and Kleekam (1993) propose that 'school culture' is manifested at three levels in the school: the transrational level, where values are based on beliefs, ethical codes and moral insights; the rational level, where values are grounded within a social context; and the subrational level, where values are experienced as personal preferences and feelings. Wyner (1991) argues that the term culture presents difficulties as well as interesting possibilities when we try to apply it to a school as a whole. Her general approach is that school culture is not only made up of unique characteristics, but is also constituted by a plurality of factors and embodies the beliefs, practices and values embedded within a school community; it is also manifested in the values, artefacts and cultural symbols valued in its community. Thus, she underscores that culture would differ from school to school. These conceptions demonstrate that 'school culture' is a complex and nuanced term with varied meanings, comprising and constituted by various factors.

Teachers are the focal point of a school and are integral in shaping its culture. The most dominant among them will be powerful in shaping its ethos, values and customs. While individuals can and will play a role in influencing school culture, the reverse can take place. School culture is shaped by, but also shapes teachers' practices in and out of school. This duality illustrates the concept's dynamic and fluid nature. Sarason's (1996) exploration of how school culture affects teachers found that it is influential in affecting relations among teachers, learners, parents, administrators and the community. It also affects how teachers define their work, how problems are solved, the way in which new ideas are implemented and how people will work together (University of Texas, 2005).

Theorists like Giroux (1981), Paquette (1991) and Popkewitz, Franklin and Pereyra (2001) regard schools as institutions of cultural and social reproduction and as a means by which society transmits its values. Giroux (1981) suggests that schooling is a contested process whereby dominant groups appropriate the school for their own ideological purposes and subordinate groups continually challenge those who are supposedly in control of them.

Bourdieu's (1993) theory of practice is useful in explaining the complex phenomenon of how schools become programmed to reproduce cultural, social and political hegemony and how they may come to be the embodiment of the community's cultural and social practices. He argues that culture embodies power relations and that intellectuals are instrumental in shaping arenas such as schools (Swartz, 1997). Bourdieu's focus is on the role culture plays in social reproduction. He defines reproduction as the strategies and processes groups pursue to produce and reproduce the conditions of their collective existence (Swartz, 1997). Culture is the key factor in enabling this reproductive process.

Understanding the general concept of culture through the lens of Bourdieu (1993), Prosser (1999), Sarason (1996), Giroux (1981), Wyner (1991), and Dalin et al (1993) helps in elucidating how schools are programmed to reproduce the community's cultural and social practices. Significantly, though, it highlights the importance of how the players in the school arena — teachers, parents and learners — contribute to and are shaped by the culture of schools.

It is difficult to understand schools, schooling and school culture in South Africa without taking into account South Africa's apartheid legacy. The apartheid regime denied black people economic and social rights, as well as access to political control. Education served as the main conduit through which such economic and social deprivation was inflicted on non-white communities. Various apartheid era education Acts entrenched segregated schooling and ensured the establishment of different education departments along racial lines, each with its own syllabi, curricula and standards of assessment; all aimed at entrenching white supremacy and the subservience of black people. Schools were often not only sites of contestation, but also of hegemonic reproduction. South Africa's apartheid legacy played a significant role in the way in which schools positioned themselves and in the way school management, teachers, parents and learners understood their roles in relation to the broader political and economic milieu. School cultures, thus, were shaped by this legacy, and continue to be so, despite 14 years of democracy. Situating school culture in its historical and political context thus becomes important in a South African context, as it explains how the legacy of apartheid played an instrumental and significant role in shaping the culture of schools.

What follows in the first part of the findings is a brief description of the schools. Here, practices that have an influence on their respective cultures are highlighted. In describing the three schools, their geographical (and economic) location, demographics, and dominant religious associations are used as key descriptors. These descriptions locate the schools in particular contexts and also help in highlighting the complexities inherent in the way schools make themselves and, importantly, how they are made by actors and practices in and outside of school.

Main findings

The findings below are presented in three parts. The first provides a context of the schools, which frames the later findings and locates the teachers within specific contexts and schools. The second is a discussion on the beliefs and practices of the teachers assessed in the study. This discussion highlights how teachers are positioned, but also how they position themselves within the specific school cultures. This description shows how their positioning reproduces unintended consequences and different sets of outcomes, often ones not intended by the official discourse of the WCED. The final section briefly describes how teachers' beliefs and the culture of schools act as filters in terms of what and how they teach, mostly in adherence to the dominant discourse of the school. *How* they do this, though, is different depending on individual agency.

Locating the schools

The description of each school below serves not only to locate the schools, but also to situate the teachers who work in these contexts. The argument made in this chapter, as will be evident in the discussion, is that teachers contribute to, but are also shaped by, the school culture, thus often making it challenging for them to reproduce a different teacher identity — eg one that is required when teaching sensitive aspects like sexuality and HIV/AIDS.

Protea Primary School

Protea Primary School is situated in an area that was designated 'Indian' by the apartheid regime, in a part of the Cape Peninsula known as the Cape Flats. The school is surrounded by 'coloured areas' and thus has a mixed population of coloured and Indian people. The community is religiously diverse, with most learners subscribing to Islam, followed by Hinduism and then Christianity.

The school comprises 280 children and nine teachers. The majority of the children and teachers live in the community. The majority of teachers are Indian, with only one black (male) teacher. Like the learners at the school, the staff are religiously diverse. Members of the community are very active in the school, with some parents selling in the tuck shop, teaching religious education, and so on.

The school prides itself on its diversity, tolerance, acceptance, community participation and family involvement. These values are exemplified through, among other things, the school principal's concern with fairness, compassion, and equality. The school's values are further exemplified when religious leaders from the community, representing Islam, Christianity and Hinduism, are invited to the school to promote tolerance, compassion, diversity and equality. There appears to be a strong belief in discipline and self-control through religion. Interestingly, there is a sense of continuity between school and community in terms of beliefs, values and practices. This could be because the principal, the chairperson of the governing body and most teachers on the staff reside within the school's community. Overall, Protea's culture may be said to be characterised by beliefs, values and practices of equality, justice, fairness, diversity, tolerance and compassion.

Highgrove Junior School

Highgrove Junior is an old school situated in an economically affluent former white suburb. It boasts a proud academic history, one that is foregrounded in many ways: through displays of excellence in the foyer and corridors, and in discussions with management. Academic success is held in high esteem, with learners not only being reminded of this at every opportunity, but also in the way learners are rewarded. The school has a learner population of 400. The school's learner population is diverse in terms of race, social status and religion. The religious affiliations of learners include Christianity, Islam, Hinduism and Judaism. Unlike the racial and religious diversity of the learners, all the teachers are Christians and all, except one, are white. The school's motto of 'Truth and Courage' is often referred to in the school. This is evident in the conduct and pedagogical practices of the principal and teachers. Although the school follows the official curriculum of the WCED at a surface level, teachers, it would seem, are more able to exercise autonomy when they need to, ie they teach content that they deem relevant even when it is not reflected in the syllabus. They were also selective about what *not* teach.

The Christian influence was evident in the way in which the school was managed. The school assembly was characterised by, among other things, the reading of verses from the Bible and the singing of Christian hymns. Christian prayers were also said. Even though many religions were represented at the school, Christianity is dominant.

Zunami Primary School

The school is situated in one of the oldest historically black townships, which forms part of the city of Cape Town's urban sprawl. The township is about 12 km from the modern, cosmopolitan city centre that attracts tourists from all over the world and also often hosts many international events. The hub of the city stands in stark contrast to this township, where poverty is visible through the type of housing and degree of unemployment. Zunami Primary is surrounded by informal settlements, with a generally transient population. All the learners and teachers are mother-tongue Xhosa speakers for whom the new democracy means little in terms of demographic and material change. An unusual feature is that, like the learners, the majority of the teachers live in the township, in close proximity to the school.

The principal's office is modest, yet adorned with photos of achievements by learners, motivational messages and messages referring to the school's ethos. The school's mission statement speaks of nurturing a holistic learner and building a learning community in which learners will find the necessary support. The school has an open-door policy where the principal is easily accessible to the staff and parents. The foyer was always abuzz with parents during all my visits to the school.

The school has a number of committees through which a sense of community is not only fostered, but also sustained. Many of the committees at school, for example, are closely aligned or responsive to the material and social needs of the immediate community. For example, the school has a bereavement committee that supports families when family members die. The school participates in prayers and other events associated with the period of bereavement, even if the death is of someone from the wider community and not closely associated with the school. It is not uncommon, therefore, to find teachers absent due to events associated with bereavement.

It was clear during observations that a blending of belief systems seems to influence relationships, teaching and classroom practices. The predominant mix appeared to be that of African traditional religious beliefs and practices with Christianity. It was confirmed in a number of interviews that traditional and Christian religious belief systems coexist complementarily and influence the school's culture and concomitant practices. The ease with which these beliefs systems are embraced as complementary plays out in the way in which teachers approach subject content, as well as in relationships among teachers themselves and between teachers and learners.

In summary, the religious influence was noticeable in all three schools, even in circumstances where the practice was one of tolerance. Another pertinent observation, especially in the two poorer schools, Zunami and Protea, was the direct influence of the community in shaping school practices. The influence of the community in the school was also evident in the way in which teachers spoke and positioned themselves — always in relation to 'their' community. Thus, it became evident — as the discussion shows later — that teachers were always aware of their community membership and this, we argue, shaped responses in and outside the classroom.

Locating the teachers: Teachers' beliefs, professional identity and reproduction of school cultures

Lesson observations revealed that the nexus between personal beliefs and school culture is complex. Often, personal beliefs acted as the dominant filter through which teachers created a professional identity in the classroom. While this may be true in the case of the majority of teachers, many were also aware of the consequences of non-adherence to the dominant community and school cultures, but chose instead to subscribe to them.

Personal beliefs and the professional practices complemented each other in the case of teachers in Zunami and Protea, where there was a close connection between school and community. The consequence of this was little conflict among the dominant school culture, teachers and teaching. Teachers often foregrounded their own beliefs in cases where these were different to, or in conflict with the dominant school culture. This, it would seem, was particularly true when their religious positions were in question. A good example in Zunami was when a male teacher suggested that his 'cultural' orientation 'forbade' him to discuss sex with children. Another teacher, whose faith forbids condom use and pre-marital sex, would not discuss safe sex options with children.

The teachers at Protea were regulated by the prevailing religious discourse in the community, whether it was Hinduism, Christianity or Islam. Values like discipline and self-control, articulated through religion, resonated in the rhetoric of Protea's ethos and the associated pedagogical practices. For example, one teacher at Protea demonstrated how Catholicism influenced the decisions he made about what to teach in Life Orientation classes. He took for granted that the principle of a union 'till death do us part', as it pertains to marriage, was part of everyone's philosophy and stated that this should not only influence the sexual decisions people make before and during marriage, but also what he is prepared to teach. Another teacher at the same school avoided using the word 'condom', because her religious principles enforced abstinence.

Like Protea, the school culture of Zunami was deeply regulated by community expectations. Teachers' work was framed within and regulated by an ideal that they often contributed to by reproducing it in their attitudes and teaching. Adherence to 'the expected' often precluded them from inserting a different discourse or giving learners alternatives with regards to, particularly, sexual choice making. For example, one teacher's facial expressions and constant comments, like 'if children should be involved with sex', expressed sentiments that suggested that children/learners had no business being sexually active. She was adamant about her position on homosexuality and showed this in her facial expressions during a class discussion. In another class discussion, a male teacher at this school gave his views on gender and the position of men in relationships; a view that was not only consistent with, but dominant in the community where the school is located. To him, men are the initiators in relationships, and they have power over females. They make choice about whom to have a relationship with and how the relationship is conducted. Once in a relationship, they also have control over women's bodies in that they often decide whether or not to discuss the use of condoms and birth control methods. This teacher was also uncomfortable with using explicit sexual terminology. Consistent with the dominant beliefs in the community, he explained that his 'culture' did not allow him to talk to children about sexual matters.

Whereas the teacher's personal and particularly religious and 'cultural' beliefs and values explicitly influenced pedagogical decisions at Protea and Zunami, the case was different with one of the observed teachers at Highgrove. This teacher positioned herself as a professional whose personal history played little role in the pedagogical choices she made. She was practised in her responses and used the utmost caution in expressing herself. By skilfully guiding the learners to lead the discussion, she tactfully avoided dealing with controversial issues and answering questions on sex, nudity and homosexuality.

What is interesting in all three schools is that teachers reproduced the dominant discourse, but in different ways. Whereas the teachers at the two other schools adhered to the dominant school culture through compliance with religious and cultural filters, the teacher at Highgrove complied through a professional position that also disallowed the insertion of a different discourse. Thus, what was evident in these schools was the degree of agency teachers exercise in influencing school culture.

Influence of school culture and teacher identity on the mediation of HIV/AIDS lessons

Approaches to, and teaching of the official content of the WCED syllabus regarding sexuality and HIV/AIDS were filtered through the relationships the teachers had with the communities in which they taught and also in the way in which they were positioned in schools (and, by implication, how they positioned themselves). Thus, and notwithstanding the above, school culture influenced teachers, shaping what was allowed or disallowed. It appeared to be powerful in conditioning teachers to be compliant, through restraint. The way it worked to produce particular teacher identities and associated classroom practices, though, was different in the respective schools.

As mentioned above, the school culture of Protea and Zunami was the embodiment of their respective communities' cultural practices and was perpetuated in the school by significant players, like teachers, principals and members of the governing body. This was evident in the committee structures and format of assemblies of the school. It was also apparent in the nature of parent involvement, namely through religious education or food preparation and school feeding schemes (particularly involving women). Highgrove's school culture, on the other hand, while also regulated, was influenced by a professional positioning that disallowed personal influences in overt ways.

School culture was also influential in determining what terminology, knowledge, perceptions, beliefs and values would be foregrounded by teachers during lessons. Teachers at the two schools displaying a close relationship with the community (Protea and Zunami) had the freedom to not only practise their beliefs safely (because the school's values were similar to their own), but to also reproduce these in particular ways in the classroom, despite it being contrary to the official curriculum of the WCED.

Protea and Zunami with their predominantly black, Indian and coloured communities, and their histories of neglect and poverty, seem to have a more established and robust relationship with their respective communities. This could be due to the fact that during the liberation struggle, these schools became sites of mobilisation, thereby establishing stronger ties with the community.

This close relationship produced particular teacher identities, with teachers making choices to reproduce dominant structures and practices consistent with those in their communities. It also enabled teachers to approach their work, particularly teaching sexuality and HIV/AIDS, from positions that were complementary to those of the community. Lessons observed were often devoid of discussion and perpetuated gender stereotypes. Constructions and expressions regarding HIV/AIDS and sexuality messages appeared to be entrenched through not only what the teachers taught, but also how they taught.

It may be concluded that such complementarity allowed for fluidity between personal and professional beliefs and values, and created a situation where personal beliefs had a more direct influence on pedagogical choices (both in terms of the content and mediation) than professional judgement. In this case, constraint on and compliance with community beliefs and values by teachers may be interpreted as voluntary, with their being aware of the consequence of non-compliance and ostracisation from the community. The corollary was that teachers made choices that were often not in the best interest of the learners and often ignored or omitted information that would enable learners to make different sexual choices or question the dominant discourse.

Regulation was felt by teachers in cases were their beliefs were in conflict with that of the school. In one case at Protea Primary School, a male teacher who lived outside the community in which the school was located felt that it was safer to comply than to go against the dominant school and, by implication, community culture. He expressed ambivalence towards using certain terminology and feared the reaction from parents if he did so, since this school's culture suggested continuity between school and community beliefs on issues of sex and sexuality. His approach would be different if he had a choice in the matter, he said. But he was silenced due to fear of the consequences that this would have for his professional career. Importantly, the school culture shaped his approach to the content and mediation process in class, thus disenabling him to convey and fulfil the curriculum requirements and, by implication, effectively preventing him from conveying appropriate HIV/AIDS information.

In the same vein, teachers at Highgrove Junior were also regulated by the school culture and displayed strict adherence to its dominant practices. The positioning by teachers, though, was very different. At this school, professionalism was privileged. The outcome of this was evident in the way in which a female teacher at this school displayed attitudes of professionalism. She constantly reminded learners of the need for correct and neat work and exercised choices that made her appear detached from the content she taught. Lessons by a male teacher at the same school also displayed similar attributes of academic excellence, objectivity for the sake of education, and professionalism. He also displayed adherence to the school motto 'Truth and Courage'. This male teacher thus foregrounded the official curriculum, despite his own strong religious beliefs about abstinence before marriage. Like his female colleague, he too encouraged discussion and allowed learners to take the lead. This was in keeping with how he understood his role as a professional. However, while the former teacher disallowed the insertion of a different discourse during class discussions, even though learners were 'involved' in producing knowledge, the latter teacher chose to discuss ways of avoiding contraction of the HI virus as dictated by the curriculum, even though these were in contradiction to his own religious beliefs (of no sex before marriage). Thus, while the process of mediation was framed by the official curriculum, the male teacher found it possible to renegotiate his professional identity, thus allowing the insertion of a discourse different to his own or that of the dominant religion(s) prevalent at the school.

In the case of Highgrove, responses to 'professionalism' took on different meanings, and compliance with a 'professional' work ethic reproduced divergent learning outcomes. In this instance, such compliance either displaced the dominant discourse or reproduced it by teachers' silences. The female teacher's silence on critical issues like condoms and homosexuality and her non-committal position, for example, indicated adherence to and reproduction of a discourse that offered learners limited alternatives, thus disregarding essential aspects of the curriculum and the school culture, despite her professionalism in other fields. In the other two schools (Protea and Zunami), where the learning outcomes remained relatively stable and teacher identities closely aligned with and relatively unchanged in relation to those of their personal identities, the learners also experienced suppression of important information about the disease, since curriculum ideology contrasted both with school and community culture and the teachers' own beliefs.

Reciprocity and the dialectic relationship between teachers and school culture

From the data, it is clear that there was a dialectic relationship and a measure of reciprocity between teachers and their respective school cultures, and that they acted iteratively to produce each other. This was evident in all instances, irrespective of the geographic location or previous racialised histories of schools. What differed, though, were the ways in which teachers drew on their own personal identities and the school culture to make a teacher identity. The way in which they did this, as the data suggests, depended primarily on the relationship schools had with their respective immediate communities.

For the most part, all the teachers in the study complied with and reproduced the dominant discourse, thus entrenching the practices and beliefs prevalent in the respective schools. In almost all instances, teachers acted with little awareness of how their actions reproduced the school culture and, in so doing, offered limited opportunities for the insertion of a different voice that would challenge practices that did not serve the interests of the learners.

Teachers' membership in the community acted as a primary filter in producing a teacher identity, particularly in cases where they either lived in the community and/or where there was a close relationship between the school and community. In such instances (particularly Protea and Zunami), teachers' personal identities often stood in the way of the professional decisions they were required to make. Thus, teachers tended to comply with and reproduce the dominant practices espoused in the community and school, blurring the distinction between the personal and professional. Teachers who felt and wanted to act differently tended to be silenced, due to fear of the consequences. The result, therefore, was also compliance with the dominant culture, even though the reasons for this were different.

Where the relationship between the school and community was less noticeable (as in the case of Highgrove Junior), teachers seemed more able to reproduce differing teacher identities that led to different learning outcomes. While they too complied with the dominant culture, it was done not only in different ways and for different reasons, but with differing consequences. At this school, teachers tended to draw on their experience of what it means to be a 'professional' to make a teacher identity. Thus, personal histories, beliefs and values, while similar to those upheld in the school, were withheld, and instead, professionalism acted as a primary filter for making a teacher identity. How this played out, though, was different in the two observed classes. At the surface level, both teachers subscribed to the official discourse of the WCED curriculum. They also both reproduced the dominant culture of the school (in this case, professionalism), but the way in which they did this was different. The male teacher observed adhered to the motto of his school, 'Truth and Courage'. However, with an emphasis on 'a professional', this teacher was able to use this position to make choices that deviated from the prescribed syllabus, which, according to him, were 'for the sake of the learners' curiosity'. According to him, he had been brought up in a culture of 'honesty and openness'; therefore, he told the children what he considered to be the truth, the facts. This was unlike the experience with the female teacher, whose uptake of professionalism resulted in silence.

The male teacher also showed how the personal and the professional coexist complementarily in spaces where autonomy and professionalism were privileged, while silences prevailed where there was a close link between community and school. In the case of the latter, personal and professional identities were blurred, resulting in silence, compliance with the dominant culture and omission of the official curriculum in the classroom.

Overall, prevailing school cultures and the ways in which teachers make their professional identities in and outside of school work iteratively to reproduce each other. In making their professional identities, they position themselves in terms of their membership of a community in and outside the school and, thus, always in relation to 'the other.' However, they did not always seem aware of the consequences that this had for what and how they taught.

Conclusion

What became clear in the study this chapter reports on was the dialectic relationship among teacher identity, community and school culture and how all worked to reproduce the 'other', but in different ways. The sensitive nature of the HIV/AIDS and sexuality content of the official syllabus resulted in teachers privileging particular positions, the consequence of which was content and mediation that offered learners information that either complied with the curriculum (foregrounding the professional identity against personal conviction) or defied it (foregrounding a deviant school/community culture and personal identity). The consequence of this is that content and mediation processes in such classrooms do not offer alternatives for learners to understand themselves and their vulnerability in relation to the HIV/AIDS pandemic.

Thus, it can be concluded that teachers of HIV/AIDS and sexuality do not always adhere to the official discourse. In fact, the official discourse as detailed in the curriculum is often undermined by the dominant school and community culture. This has serious implications for intervention strategies in schools and the achievement of intended objectives.

Chapter 5

Aysha Hattas
University of Cape Town

Examining Religious Leaders' and Traditional Healers' Responses to HIV/AIDS in a Modern Community

Introduction

Certain individuals, such as teachers, sports personalities and religious leaders, often serve as models that the general population looks to for guidance on issues such as prevention of new infections, sexuality, supporting the infected, etc. Often, religious leaders and traditional healers[1] are particularly influential in that they act as the moral conscience of society, specifying the norms to which societies should adhere (Ahmed, 1999). They hold positions that are looked upon as authoritative and are associated with having direct links to the divine or supreme being. They are often called upon to render counselling or advice on ethical, moral and behavioural issues affecting the societies in which they live. In some instances, they use holy scriptures to give advice, and in other instances, they offer healing through the use of traditional medicines or prayer.

As role models, and unlike other personalities in positions of influence, religious leaders are usually in direct communication with their respective communities on a regular basis. As such, it is often assumed that they have knowledge and an understanding of the complexities of daily life in ways that other leaders might not. Thus, they have the ability to influence the individual and collective identities of societies (Hewson, 1998).

Religious leaders and healers are also viewed as those who may provide solace to people during periods of vulnerability. For example, in societies that have experienced natural disasters or where the threat of disease impacts on their daily lives, as in the case of HIV/AIDS today. Sometimes their advice and responses to issues can be contradictory or out of touch with the realities and experiences of members of their communities.

Religious leaders are often called upon by governments to assist in the promotion of healthy lifestyles. Such a request was made by the government to religious leaders in South Africa to assist in combating the increasing rates of HIV infection. In 1999 the South African Department of National Education, through its National Education Policy for HIV/AIDS, proposed that all learners, teachers and communities be educated about HIV/AIDS. This policy proposed collaboration between HIV/AIDS units in departments of education and faith-based organisations in this regard.

1 The term 'traditional healers' is used synonymously with 'sangoma' or 'spiritual healers'. On occasion, respondents are referred to as 'leaders and healers', or 'religious leaders', or simply as 'leaders'.

As a pandemic that is transmitted primarily through sexual contact, HIV/AIDS forces religious leaders and healers to confront the deeply private issues of sex and sexuality in public spaces not usually associated with such discourses. While in their private capacities, leaders and healers may subscribe to their own personal beliefs on sex and disease, in their public roles they are required to make 'professional' judgements using religion and morality as a frame of reference.

This chapter raises questions about how religious leaders and traditional healers are positioned and how they position themselves in relation to the pandemic. It asks questions about their attitudes, responses and experiences of the disease and how discourses of sex and sexuality influence their experiences of and responses to the pandemic. The chapter also examines ways in which these leaders and healers navigate their way between religion and disease in community contexts where modern[2] and traditional discourses exist.

Methodology

The study this chapter reports on was located within a qualitative research approach as it was mainly concerned with understanding rather than explaining social action. It utilised phenomenological and narrative approaches. The phenomenological approach was used as it recognises that people are constantly in the process of constructing, developing and shifting their daily life patterns, which in turn alters their experiences (Babbie & Mouton, 2001). It provided a framework for the study to trace how people (specifically religious leaders) have constructed and reconstructed their responses to disease and how they have positioned themselves in their respective communities.

The narrative approach was utilised mainly to provide a script — a story — about religious leaders' experiences regarding HIV/AIDS, both from a personal and professional perspective. Narratives help show how people make meaning for themselves. Thus, in telling their stories, religious leaders and traditional healers made available rich data that was thick with descriptions. These descriptions provided the study with insights into the contexts in which the leaders operate on a daily basis, sketching for the researcher the scripts/stories of their lives.

Sampling

The study utilised both random and purposive sampling techniques. All the primary schools in the Cape Metropole area were clustered according to the racial categories[3] that were used during the apartheid era, ie prior to 1994. From these schools, five were randomly selected.

The five selected schools were used as a basis for accessing religious leaders. The principals provided insights into the various religious communities represented in the schools and also directed me to religious sites such as mosques, churches and synagogues near the schools. A sample of 18 religious leaders, ie three traditional heal-

[2] A modern community is defined by Iverson Software (2005:1) as 'a community with a relatively complex division of labour, whose inhabitants tend to welcome change, use sophisticated technology, have well-developed mass media, and rely more on formal, secondary relationships than on primary or informal relationships'.

[3] That is, 'white', 'Indian', 'coloured' and 'black' schools.

ers, two Jewish leaders, four Christian leaders, three Muslim leaders and six Rastafarian leaders, was purposively selected.

Because of the sensitive nature of the research, respondents were assured of their confidentiality, and are referred to using pseudonyms in this chapter (see Table 5.1).

Table 5.1: Respondents

Traditional healers	Jewish leaders	Christian leaders	Muslim leaders	Rastafarian leaders
Mamela	Rabbi P	Pastor Allen	Imama Fatima	Elder Job
Tando	Rabbi O	Priest Brian	Moulana Omar	Elder Aaron
Chiko		Pastor Jeff	Imam Ali	Elder Solomon
		Priest Ted		Elder David
				Elder Ezra
				Elder Bianca

Methods of data collection

Data for the study was collected using in-depth interviews, focus group discussions (FGDs) and observations. Initial informal visits to the respective religious sites were followed by formal meetings for interviews, FGDs or observations. In-depth interviews provided insight into the private and personal lives of the respondents.

FGDs were conducted with two groups: Rastafarian elders and Christian leaders. The FGDs elicited information about their experiences, thoughts and knowledge regarding HIV/AIDS. Observations occurred while the religious leaders were teaching in their places of worship or at the sample schools where they taught. This method allowed me to examine the leaders in their domains and in relation to their congregants or learners. In the case of traditional healers, confidentiality constraints did not allow me to observe entire healing sessions. On one occasion, however, I observed the end portion of an interactive session between the healer and a patient.

Sensitivity to the context

As a researcher, access to the religious leaders was dependent on adherence to the codes and regulations of the various religious communities. This meant that I had to adhere to particular dress codes, and in some instances I had to be accompanied by my husband. In the latter cases, it was because in these communities, men (the religious leaders) were not allowed to be alone in a private space with an unfamiliar woman. I acknowledge that these sensitivities and my identity as a woman, may have an impact on what religious leaders were prepared to disclose.

Theoretical framework

Durkheim's conception of religion and its role in structuring society is used to inform the analysis of the findings. Durkheim understands religion as the nucleus of society and sees it as an important constituent that holds communities together. By defining religion as a 'unified system of beliefs and practices relative to sacred things, things set apart and surrounded by prohibitions — beliefs and practices that unite its adherents in a single moral community called a church' (in Cosman, 2001:46), Durkheim places religion at the core of all social life and, as such, its ultimate role is to act as a guide for people (in Binsbergen, 2003). He contends that religion is important for communities because of its cohesive function, and that it is 'not divinely or supernaturally inspired', but rather a creation of society that is 'eminently social… [and consists of] collective representations' (Durkheim in Cosman, 2001:46). To him, religion conveys shared aspects and truths that belong to the community. The role of religion, therefore, is to stimulate, sustain or recreate people's ways of thinking within a particular society and, as such, maintain social cohesion. Any issues to be dealt with in the community are approached in a way that is common to all, as 'religious facts, as social affairs and the product of collective thought' (Durkheim in Cosman, 2001:46).

According to Durkheim, religious life is divided into different spheres, which he refers to as the 'sacred and profane' (Durkheim, 2001:159). Sacred refers to all the spiritual aspects of life and includes rituals, symbols and places of worship. In adherence to these, people draw strength and obtain direction in both the physical and moral aspects of their lives. Profane, on the other hand, indicates anything else that does not hold religious significance. This includes routine behaviour, daily work and domestic duties, and is essentially that which occurs outside ritualised periods of religious adherence.

Berger (1977) and Rohmann (2002), in line with Durkheim (1952), state that the position of religion shifted at the onset of the scientific revolution during the 17th century. Rohmann (2002:265) argues that modernity rejected traditional and conventional forms of life in the quest to foster innovation and new empirical foundations. Modernity was perceived as being inherently advanced in relation to whatever preceded it, including concepts of religion and tradition. The findings of the present study question whether modernity has displaced the discursive space in which religious leaders operate beyond the religious domain. This study advances a theory that distinguishes and differentiates the ways in which religious leaders position themselves in the context of modernity.

The relationship between religion and disease, as discussed by Foucault (in Cousins & Hussain, 1985), Allen (2000; 2001) and Sontag (1989), also provides important conceptual tools for this study. Foucault (in Cousins & Hussain, 1985) contends that historically, the way in which people, especially religious leaders, interpreted diseases led to particular responses. Foucault (in Cousins & Hussain, 1985) and Allen (2001) argue that when people were unsure about the reasons why diseases occurred, they turned to religion for answers. Allen (2001) further explains that while people were unsure, so too were the religious leaders they turned to, especially in the absence of scientific evidence. As a result, people, including religious leaders, resorted to speculation about the origin of a particular disease, as well as the reasons for its occurrence.

Foucault (in Cousins & Hussain, 1985) and Allen (2001) state that the interpretations given by leaders often held negative connotations, since they saw disease as the result of people engaging in immoral and irreligious behaviours. Thus, historically, the understanding of disease has foregrounded moral interpretations in which people's behaviour came under scrutiny rather than emphasising the need for physical healing. Some religious teachings still understand and interpret certain diseases, especially those that are transmitted mainly through sexual intercourse, from a moral perspective (Paasche-Orlow & Rosenn, 2001; Abdul-Wahhab, 2001; Thanvi, 1992; Goss, 2001). These teachings emphasise that there is a relationship between disease and immoral behaviour.

Overall, as a modern disease, HIV/AIDS brings together discourses of religion, disease and sexuality in distinct ways, emphasising how the complex social context presents new challenges for religious leaders and healers.

Main findings

The findings of the study suggest that there is no single response to the way in which religious leaders and healers understand and respond to HIV/AIDS. Responses showed agreement and disagreement both within and across religions, and highlighted the inherent tensions that resulted from trying to maintain traditional religious practices, on the one hand, and responding to specific contexts, on the other.

What emerged in the findings are two religious discourses that I refer to as either 'closed' or 'open'. The discussion is given depth by the tensions that arise within these two discourses. A 'closed' religious discourse is characterised by its scriptural base, conservatism, a moral position, adherence to tradition and resistance to change. It places emphasis on a collective identity and the role of 'traditional religious leaders' in directing the process. Contrastingly, the open discourse, while also adhering to basic religious principles, is more amendable and fluid in regards to discussions and responses to special issues and concerns that arise in the context of HIV/AIDS.

Religion and the place and purpose of sex

Responses to HIV/AIDS cannot be separated from the complex views that people have about religion, disease, infection and sex and the connections among these. Importantly, the responses of the group of religious leaders (those involved in the study), could not be removed from the place and purpose of sex in social life. The discussion that follows, therefore, focuses on these responses.

All the leaders, with the exception of the sangomas, said that the primary purpose of sex was procreation and the preservation of the sanctity of life. Procreation was functional and not necessarily always associated with pleasure or sexual indulgence. Sex, however, was only acceptable in the context of marriage or long-term, stable relationships. For example, Rabbi O stressed that sex was a necessary part of marriage and its main purpose was procreation, especially within religious families. This view was echoed by Rabbi P, who explained that sex is the means through which God's requirements are met and sustained. Ultimately, the belief was that 'life belongs to God; it is a blessing'. Here Rabbi P referred to the Jewish father figure, 'Father Abraham', who had many sons, and therefore all Jews ought to aspire to having many children — but, of course, within the context of marriage.

The Muslim leaders also agreed that sex was for procreation and should occur within the context of marriage. Christian leaders concurred with this thinking: 'When you get married, what is the initial idea of having sex? It's having children, wanting a family, carrying on my name, that's why I've got boys', Pastor Allen argued. While the Rastafarians did not believe in conventional marriages, they did, however, believe in long-term and stable relationships. It is in this context that they believed sex should occur.

Two responses in this group of people were prominent: firstly, that sex was for procreation and, secondly, that sex should only occur in the context of marriage. Understanding the way religious leaders viewed sex is important, as these views directly influenced the way in which they developed their positions about HIV/AIDS as a sexually transmitted disease, and how they interpreted its transmission. Since the dominant position of the religious leaders was that sex should only occur in the context of marriage and only for procreation, this positively correlated with the moralist view that sexually transmitted diseases were a consequence of immoral and irreligious behaviour (Foucault in Cousins & Hussain, 1985; Allen, 2001).

Working with the views expressed above, it could be said that a 'closed' religious discourse shapes the religious leaders' opinions on the place and purpose of sex, where sex is understood as being for the purpose for procreation, that pleasure was not necessarily a part of the sexual experience, and that sex should occur exclusively within the context of marriage. These findings are synonymous with Bullough and Bullough's (1994:514) argument that religious leaders regard sex in terms of a 'fixed world view'.

However, this traditional discourse is at odds with modernity and reality. By this I mean that religious leaders respond in the way that they do because their frame of reference is a traditional religious one that is based on a literal reading of religious scriptures (Paasche-Orlow & Rosenn, 2001; Abdul-Wahhab, 2001; Thanvi, 1992; Goss, 2001). This perspective ignores the fact that people live in a modern society with modern challenges such as HIV/AIDS. According to Menka (2005) and Allott (1999), the encouragement of a traditional perspective does not account for the reality that people do engage in sex, procreate and have families outside marriage (Menka, 2005).

Views on transmission, sexual behaviour and risk

All the respondents agreed that HIV was transmitted primarily through sexual contact, be it 'deviant' behaviour or not. All respondents were also aware that there were other forms of transmission that included, among others, blood transfusions.

All the Muslim respondents were of the opinion that infection occurred primarily through promiscuity, extra-marital sexual relationships and as a result of 'going against nature' through 'deviant' sexual practices. Two of the Muslim leaders believed that transmission took place mainly through 'illicit sex [and] homosexual sex', or, as the third one emphasised, adults 'sleeping around', specifically 'married men and women'. Consistent with their views on the place and function of sex, the three Muslim leaders situated transmission in the context of sexual behaviour that goes against traditional religious beliefs and norms.

Not unlike the religious leaders, Mamela, a traditional healer (sangoma), argued that HIV was spread 'mainly through sexual immorality'. She was aware of infidelity in the communities that she served and its contribution to the spread of the disease. Mamela also pointed out that in the case of married people, it was difficult for the partners to negotiate the use of condoms as protection, since marriage was seen as an institution where there were only two supposedly faithful partners, thus eliminating the need for the use of condoms. Mamela also lamented the compromised position of women, which often made it difficult for them to negotiate safe sex practices in marriage.

The Christian leaders, while acknowledging that the most common way of contracting HIV was through sex, also indicated knowledge of other ways of transmission, such as through infected blood. Regarding transmission through sex, Pastor Brian blamed this on homosexuality, rape and indulgence with 'different sexual partners'. The Christian leaders lamented that teenagers were potentially at risk of infection, among other things, because of having multiple sexual partners. Overall, the Christian leaders were concerned that sex was taking place outside of the 'safe' confines of marriage.

The two Jewish leaders also indicated knowledge of the various ways in which HIV was transmitted, ie through sex, blood transfusions, sharing of unsterilised needles (especially by drug abusers) and mother to child transmission. The rabbis also pointed out that medical doctors were at high risk of infection because of the nature of their work. An interesting observation by the rabbis (especially Rabbi O) was that Jews were less at risk of contracting HIV/AIDS through sex, and were more likely to contract HIV through contact with contaminated blood, as in the case of doctors in the course of their work. Implicit in this view is the notion that Jews were less promiscuous and, therefore, less vulnerable to infection by HIV/AIDS through sex. This view also points towards the notion of invulnerability to HIV infection by Jews.

The Rastafarian leaders denied that HIV infection was ever possible in their communities. Elder Bianca stated that 'HIV is never something that I have "seen" amongst us. It's very scarce. I don't know any Rasta that has that disease'. Elder Bianca claimed that HIV/AIDS did not exist in her community because, as a religious group, members were protected by the practice of smoking a 'holy' herb called 'Ghanja'. She explained:

> Ghanja plays a big role amongst Rastas ... our blood is full of Ghanja. Ghanja protects us from any disease ... Ghanja in your blood; it's not easy for any disease to attack you. It warms your blood and kills other things before they get in.

The belief that Ghanja, an illegal intoxicant in many countries, could protect Rastafarians from contracting HIV/AIDS could in fact predispose them to HIV infection.

The belief of Rabbi O and the Rastafarians that their communities were not at risk of HIV infection is not consistent with available evidence, which shows that HIV/AIDS infects all communities irrespective of religion, race or sex (UNAIDS, 2005). This study perceives such denial as a 'tension coping mechanism' or as a means to avoid confrontations arising from the shift in communities' traditional practices. This means that people no longer conform to traditional practices; instead, they are informed by their individual choices, which may not necessarily be aligned with traditional patterns. Furthermore, the study suggests that the above denial stems from an authoritative religious voice, which leads communities to the belief that HIV/AIDS does not affect them. The consequence of such a belief is that people in these communities may not fight the disease or attempt to employ preventive measures when they adhere to the authoritative voices in their communities. It would seem that the authoritative voices, in this instance, may negatively impact on the suggested 'open' discourse that would allow for discussion around the use of improved preventive measures.

Vulnerability and risk

Although Rastafarian respondents disputed that their followers could contract the virus, they gave what they thought were the reasons for the high HIV/AIDS prevalence in South Africa. All six Rastafarians agreed that poverty was the main reason for the escalation in HIV prevalence. Elder Bianca argued that there was a link between poverty and vulnerability, especially among women. She said:

> When you're poor you're at a disadvantage. For women, it is easier than for men to catch [HIV]. [Say] I am a woman with children ... [and] don't have anything to eat. I'll have sex with him, deal with him, I give my life away. Poverty is the cause.

Elder Aaron concurred with Elder Bianca's view that women were forced to use their bodies for economic gain. He gave the example of young girls having children with old men to illustrate this point. On his part, Elder Ezra felt that economic conditions played a role in determining access to condoms. He further claimed that condoms were related to HIV infection. He explained:

> ... condoms are in different classes, different grades, a local one or expensive one. The rich man survive using the expensive one, the poor don't survive because he uses the cheap one. I find the cheap one spreads AIDS amongst the poor.

While poverty was considered to be a key condition that encouraged the spread of the disease, one respondent among the Rastafarian group offered reasons that had little to do with socioeconomic conditions. Elder Aaron felt that condoms encouraged promiscuity, particularly by married women. He stated: 'We're saying no you don't need condoms; it says yes you can do adultery.' It is unclear why Elder Aaron thought that condom use encouraged adultery especially by married women and not men.

Similar views on the link between condom use and risky sexual behaviour were expressed by Pastor Jeff, who also felt that the promotion of condom use encouraged extra-marital sex. The other Christian leaders linked infection and vulnerability more directly to sin and punishment. According to them, infections were the result of choices people make to sin, rather than the result of external influences such as poverty. The consequences, therefore, were infection, which was interpreted as punishment for sinful and 'deviant' sexual behaviour such as homosexuality, incest or extra-marital relationships. Pastor Allen, for example, suggested the following explanation:

> ... in the Old Testament Solomon had 700 wives but there was nothing like AIDS then. Somewhere along God has made up his mind and said enough is enough and allowed this [HIV]. He allowed it because people wouldn't listen. Jesus said that you shall love the Lord your God, and love your own wife. ... they [people] started mixing it and now [they are] having sex with their daughters, and this is where God has just had it.

The Muslim leaders also linked sin to HIV/AIDS infection. Engaging in sex outside of marriage was considered sinful, and so was homosexuality. They felt that sex within marriage provided one with protection from HIV/AIDS. Infection was therefore interpreted as punishment from God, although people born with HIV/AIDS were not seen as being punished by God.

The Rabbis had conflicting views on vulnerability and risk. For Rabbi O, infection was not a concern. To him, contraction of HIV was linked to 'pre-marital sex, which is [a] sin', and he felt that Jews were not promiscuous, and thus not vulnerable to infection. He said, 'it is a problem, but it doesn't seem to me to be an enormous problem in the Jewish community'. Rabbi P, on the other hand, differentiated between promiscuity and risky sexual behaviour. To him, infection with HIV depended on how responsibly people behaved rather than on whether or not they were promiscuous.

The sangomas concurred that infection was related to sinful practices. However, unlike the Jewish, Christian and Muslim leaders, 'sin' was perceived as the *consequences* of the sexual act rather than the *act* itself. Sangoma Mamela suggested that infection was 'due to sexual immorality and infidelity'. She offered clients condoms as a means of protection, because she 'didn't want sins with God'. 'Sins with God' meant that she did not want to participate in abortions and deaths, which were consequences of sex. Having sex, therefore, was not necessarily sinful, but it could lead to sin, hence the provision and encouragement of the use of condoms.

Sangoma Chiko's explanation for contracting HIV was based on a cultural practice that discouraged the use of condoms: 'There's no way you can sleep with a woman with a condom; traditional men won't condomise.' The belief was that procreation was more important than protection against disease. According to him, men who use condoms would be stereotyped as not being 'real men'. Chiko, however, recognised the importance of condom use as a preventive measure.

All the sangomas claimed that they advocated condom use because people engaged in sex at younger ages, and that they feared that many young people would lose their lives due to HIV/AIDS. Sangoma Tando said: 'Before they'd do those things [sex] when they're older, today they do sex at young ages. That's why they're suffering more from venereal diseases.' Sangoma Mamela added that previously the youth would experiment with sex through mock sex, but presently they engage in 'direct intercourse'. Therefore, she encouraged condom use as protection against infection.

Imama Fatima also advocated condom use. Her encouragement of condom use followed the death of her friend from HIV/AIDS: 'She was only 14. She was so young and yes, sexually active at that age.' However, she advocated condom use as a last resort, after abstinence. The Christian leaders, like the other leaders, acknowledged that the youth were more at risk of HIV/AIDS infection. Two of the Christian leaders explained youth vulnerability to HIV/AIDS infection along racial lines. Pastor Jeff alluded to the idea that 'the non-white society' was more at risk. Pastor Brian put it thus: 'White learners [are] sheltered about sex issues. Coloured and blacks are more outgoing; they're sleeping around in grade eight and nine. Whites start sex in matric, grade 11, at varsity.' Like the sangomas and Imama Fatima, Pastor Brian, too, argued for condom use by the youth.

As evidenced above, conceptions of vulnerability and risk varied across and within religions. Other than the Rastafarians and one of the rabbis who considered their communities as not being at risk of HIV/AIDS infection, all the other leaders acknowledged that their communities were vulnerable to infection by the disease. Generally, the religious leaders and sangomas seemed to concur that women and the youth were the groups most vulnerable to infection by HIV/AIDS.

Of paramount concern for this study were the responses of the Rastafarian and Muslim leaders regarding vulnerability to HIV/AIDS infection by their communities. The Rastafarian leaders limited their communities' vulnerability to reasons of poverty, particularly blaming poverty for exposing women to sexual exploitation. Their views, however, underplayed the reality that Rastafarian men are allowed to engage in polygamous relationships and that condom use is not permitted because of the religious prescription that procreation cannot be restricted.

Similar to the views of the Rastafarian leaders, Muslim leaders also associated vulnerability to and contraction of HIV/AIDS with engagement in 'deviant' and 'immoral' sexual behaviour. However, within this religion, men are also allowed to enter into polygamous marriages, which present possibilities for infections, especially in light of adherence to the Muslim religious law that prohibits the use of condoms. Within these two religious groups, it is apparent that women are more vulnerable to HIV/AIDS infection than men because they may become infected in a polygamous relationship or because they are the ones that engage in prostitution for a living, especially young Rastafarian girls.

The risk of infection by women in Muslim polygamous marriages is further evidenced by the fact that whereas the incoming wife (the second, third, etc) was expected to take an HIV/AIDS test, the same was not required of her husband. This emphasised a 'closed' religious discourse that perpetuates male dominance and ignores the reality of female vulnerability.

Disease prevention strategies and religious beliefs

All the sangomas and religious leaders, with the exception of Rabbi O, acknowledged that their communities were vulnerable to HIV/AIDS infection. Present in the discussions on preventive strategies was the use of condoms. As has previously been alluded to, eleven of the eighteen leaders perceived condom use as a mechanism that prevented procreation, which apparently goes against the primary religious function of sex. Other responses included the perception that condoms were a means of discarding lives and an interference with the natural processes of people 'meeting and cohabitating'.

The leaders gave alternative preventive strategies and also explained why condom use was discouraged by their religions. Rastafarians believed that if the South African government alleviated poverty, then HIV/AIDS would be prevented. They were also of the opinion that the quality of condoms was related to the increase in infections. To them, discarding condom use was a strategy for HIV/AIDS prevention.

While Rabbi O indicated that he might encourage the use of condoms as the very last resort, Rabbi P focused on the notion of saving sperm, which Rabbi O also alluded to. He (Rabbi P) echoed the Torah: 'The seed of man was limited so you don't want to waste seed … so condom use is prohibited because you are sending a message that you don't want life.' Rabbi P also advocated the use of condoms in some instances. He argued that life was complex and therefore in certain instances he would advocate condom use.

Imama Fatima, while supporting the use of condoms as a last resort, insisted that abstinence was the best way to avoid HIV/AIDS. She also advised that 'getting married the moment you have feelings for a person' was yet another way of preventing HIV/AIDS infection. The other Muslim leaders disagreed with Imama Fatima's views on the use of condoms, believing that condom use was not a strategy for prevention of HIV/AIDS infection.

Two Christian priests insisted that people should abstain from sex until they were married. Pastor Brian posited that 'we wouldn't be dealing with the crisis of HIV/AIDS if people chose [not] to have sex out of the covenant of marriage'. As for condoms, Pastor Brian argued: 'As far as I'm aware, there is no reference to the use of condoms [in the Bible], but there are a lot of principles in the Bible that we can live by.' However, Pastor Brian, like Imama Fatima, felt that condoms could be used in some instances.

Consistent with the stance against condom use by the Rastafarian leaders, Rastafarian Bianca agreed with the Rabbis about not spilling sperm, but disagreed with them about abstinence. She argued that she could not dictate to people when they should have sex. She said: 'It's not right to put your sperm in a bubble and throw it into garbage, and it's not right to tell people not to have sex; it's natural.' Therefore, condoms were not an option for her and neither was abstinence a prevention strategy.

The three sangomas claimed that they advocated the use of condoms as a prevention strategy.

As the foregoing analysis shows, the various religious frames of reference act as the lens through which religious leaders position themselves and interpret religious principles. The leaders are generally strict. Their interpretation of religious principles creates different degrees of tension between their beliefs and the reality and challenges experienced in communities. The result is that the messages they transmit regarding HIV/AIDS are either 'closed' or 'open', depending on the degree of compliance with the dominant discourse of that particular religion.

Discussion

The above analysis shows the interplay of the 'open' and 'closed' discourses, even though the 'closed' discourse appears to be more prominent. The data shows that most religious leaders in the study were still very conservative and advocated an adherence to traditional religious principles, especially with regard to sex and condom use. They maintained that sex was only allowed in the context of marriage, meaning that premarital sex was a sin and its consequences were a punishment from God. The leaders also claimed that condom use encouraged promiscuity and also interfered with the primary religious purpose of sex, which was procreation.

Most religious leaders position sex within the confines of a 'fixed world view' (Bullough & Bullough, 1994:514). This is the result of a literal reading of religious scriptures, despite the fact that people are living in a modern society with modern challenges such as HIV/AIDS. According to Menka (2005) and Allott (1999), and as shown in this study, the encouragement of traditional adherence ignores the reality that people engage in sex outside of marriage and not necessarily for procreation. Thus, the discouragement of condom use by religious leaders inadvertently promotes the conditions for HIV infections to occur. The same applies to notions of invulnerability held by the Rastafarians and the Orthodox Jewish rabbi. Such notions, coupled with condemnation of condom use, can be said to be a recipe for an increase in HIV infections.

The 'closed' religious discourse in which strict adherence to the formal religious texts is encouraged creates tension in considering the use of condoms. As Berger (1997) explains, people can exercise the choice of when to use condoms; ie having sex for the purpose of procreation or for pleasure. In his view, the reasons for having sex and also condom use have become a matter of personal decision and choice. Such choices have resulted in tensions for religious leaders who wish to oversee the execution of rigid religious principles within communities that are making choices outside of religious boundaries.

The 'closed' religious discourse is also in conflict with the HIV/AIDS prevention strategies that are being implemented. Although most of these strategies advocate abstinence, they also promote condom use, but it is unlikely that conservative religious leaders would support the latter strategy. This has implications for the success of such programmes, given the influence of religious leaders in society. Overall, the 'closed' religious discourse was rigid, advocated strict adherence to scripture that determined 'moral' uprightness and seemed to condemn those who are infected with HIV/AIDS as being punished for sin.

In contrast to the 'closed' religious discourse, some religious leaders can be said to adhere to an 'open' religious discourse. As already mentioned, the 'open' religious discourse adheres to basic religious principles, but is flexible and advocates an adaptation, to some extent, to modern challenges. Therefore, this discourse takes into account the reality of the challenges facing communities and the anxieties created by these challenges, where, for example, as the data indicates, more people are engaging in sexual activity at younger ages than in traditional times. This, together with the understanding that religion intends to preserve life, is important to these leaders, therefore, their responses were different from those who hold more conservative views. In this study, these are defined as traditional modern leaders who understand the complex interplay between tradition and modernity, and who recognise these as coexisting with each other rather than in parallel. For instance, they encouraged people to use condoms as a means of protection.

Only the sangomas, two Christians, one Muslim and one Jewish leader could be said to be such traditional modern leaders. While a minority group in the study, they did provide evidence of the complex changing religious space and how, within it, modernity and tradition come together to produce and reproduce a different discourse. Unlike the 'closed' religious discourse that often positioned HIV/AIDS outside the formal religious space, thus disallowing any discussion of its consequences, the 'open' religious discourse allowed for transformations of perceptions of HIV/AIDS and was more in line with many HIV/AIDS prevention strategies. This 'open' religious discourse, like many HIV/AIDS prevention strategies, first encouraged abstinence, but also viewed condom use as being helpful in combating the disease.

Conclusion

The study set out to examine the responses and experiences of religious leaders and traditional healers to HIV/AIDS within a modern community. It is apparent that these people were situated in a complex position, wedged between their traditional religious beliefs and practices, and modern challenges such as HIV/AIDS. From the analysis, it is evident that religious leaders had potential to influence the way people thought about religion and contentious issues such as HIV/AIDS.

As was pointed out above, two discourses emerged, a 'closed' religious discourse and an 'open' religious discourse. The former, which is distinguished by its adherence to tradition, a narrow view of morality and strict adherence to religious scriptures, epitomises a religious discourse that offers limited possibilities for change or the adjustment of lifestyles to modern realities. Some of the religious leaders who subscribed to this discourse saw the threat of HIV/AIDS as less of a problem in their respective communities and tended to 'other' its impact. Condom use was discouraged, since it was often associated with promiscuous or immoral behaviour. Those subscribing to the latter, 'open', discourse, while still adhering to basic religious principles, were more amenable to modern initiatives, such as condom use, to prevent infection. They thus subsumed the social challenges that people face in a modern community in the wake of HIV/AIDS into their religious frameworks.

Therefore, the chapter thus argues that whereas the 'closed' discourse could encourage further HIV/AIDS infections, the 'open' discourse could contribute towards combating the disease.

PART 3

YOUTH, IDENTITY, SEXUALITY AND HIV/AIDS

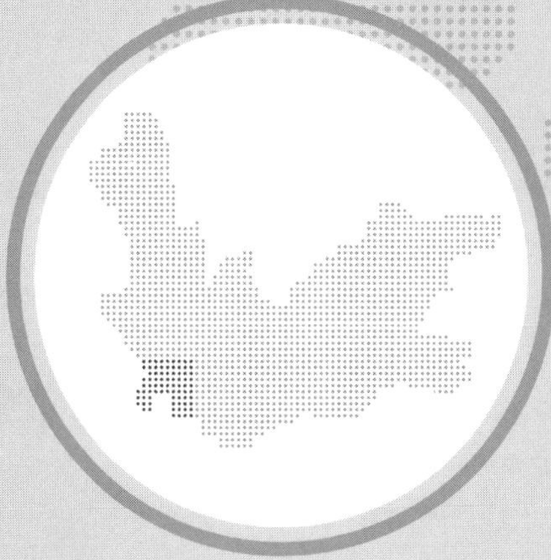

CAPE TOWN

Chapter 6

Hilda Rolls
University of Cape Town

Masculinising and Feminising Identities: Factors Shaping Primary School Learners' Sexual Identity Construction in the Context of HIV/AIDS

Introduction

Childhood is, by definition, a complex phenomenon. It is perceived in different ways and comes with a variety of explanations and interpretations. Mead and Wolfentstein (in Jenks, 1996:60) argue that childhood is a phenomenon that was, until the onset of modernity, taken for granted. It was seen as 'a figure of speech, a mythological subject rather than a subject of articulate scrutiny'. Over the last 100 years, understandings of childhood have shifted from those that accorded the child a minimal sense of recognition to more contemporary understandings that have begun to encompass an understanding that children have rights that are no different from, and, in some senses, even greater than those of adults. Much of this change has come about as a result of notions of identity that have moved from essentialist biologism to more social notions seeking to be more holistic (James, Jenks & Prout, 1998).

Several perspectives have been advanced to try and account for the ways in which children develop, and construct their identities. Such perspectives have been developed by theorists such as Jean Piaget, Kohlberg, Sigmund Freud and Erik Erikson (Shilling, 1993; Lemner & Badenhorst, 1997; Corsaro, 1997; Cole & Cole, 2001; Woodward, 2002). The upsurge in the incidence of HIV/AIDS and the increasing involvement of children in sex have played important roles in generating more interest in children's sexual identity construction. More attention, therefore, needs to be focused on children as they attempt to use their agency and are being shaped by the social contexts within which they find themselves (James et al, 1998).

This chapter is drawn from a study that explored ways in which ten-year-old children constructed their sexual identities within the South African HIV/AIDS context. According to Parker (1995), there is a paucity of theory about human sexuality in general. He attributes this to the naturalist viewpoint of sexuality that has played an influential role in AIDS research thus far. Interestingly, Parker foregrounds the issue of context by explaining that 'sexual desire has been treated, in many ways as a kind-of-given, and the social and cultural factors shaping sexual experience in different settings have largely been ignored' (Parker, 1995:261). Scant as our understanding might be of sexuality in our wider social world, it is even more so in the case of child sexuality. Given this line of logic, especially as regards the understanding of sexuality in the context of HIV/AIDS, this chapter explores how sexual identities are constructed and reconstructed by ten-year-old children in some primary schools in the Western Cape Province, South Africa.

A major concern of the chapter is whether the environment in which children are growing up provides an atmosphere that contributes positively to their sexual identity construction. The basic premise of this chapter centres on notions of identity as socially constructed in complex contexts that are, in the case of South Africa, deeply racialised and gendered. From such a perspective, children's growth and development cannot be understood outside the social practices in which they constitute and make meaning of their lives.

Methodology

As the study was aimed at investigating how children constructed their sexual identities, a methodological approach that prioritised the subjective experience and perspective of the child was appropriate (Greig & Taylor, 1999). A qualitative approach was therefore used, since it allowed for particular attention to be paid to children's responses and experiences within a naturalistic context. Within this paradigm, human action is viewed from the point of view of the social participants themselves and their specific responses to a social phenomenon in which they are participants (Babbie et al, 2001).

Sampling

The sampling of schools involved in the study proceeded as follows. All primary schools in the Cape Metropolitan area were categorised into the four pre-1994 racialised system of schools, ie white, Indian, coloured and black schools. One school was then randomly selected from each of the four groups, except for previously black schools, from which two schools were randomly selected. Thus, five schools were selected for the study.

Table 6.1 shows the total number of children selected, as well as the different data collection strategies used in the study.

Table 6.1: Data collection strategies and study sample

Data collection strategy	Sample of learners	Total number of learners
1. Questionnaire survey	Entire gr. 5 class in each school	Average: 25–35 learners per school
2. Focus group interviews	Selected 8–12 mixed gender groups at each school	8–12 learners per school
3. Individual interviews	5 learners from each school	5 learners per school
4. Observations	Learners' behaviour in class-room and on playground	25–35 learners per school; playground, depending on activity; eg skipping rope: 8 learners

Methods of data collection

As shown in Table 6.1, several methods of data collection were utilised. These included observations, questionnaires, focus group discussions and individual interviews.

Observations were conducted at school and took two forms — those in the classroom and on the playground. Since the study was concerned with sexual identity construction, the children were observed during Life Orientation lessons. Outside the classroom, attention was paid to how children occupied their free time and how they interacted with one another.

To understand the socioeconomic characteristics of the children, all the learners in the selected classes completed a questionnaire. The results from the questionnaire were used as a guide in the selection of between 8–12 children from each of the five designated classes for the focus group discussions. Consideration was given to the manner in which they responded to the variables of parental status, home environment and economic status. Five children from each focus group were selected for individual interviews.

Analysis was ongoing throughout the period of data collection, due to the sequential nature of the data collection process and the reliance on results from one set of instruments for the development of the next.

Sensitivity to the topic and working with children

Two issues were pertinent in selecting data collection tools for the study, ie the sensitivity of the topic and challenges around working with children. Sexuality is a sensitive topic and the researcher therefore had to be sensitive to the topic. Questions were asked in a 'non-embarrassing' manner and sensitive questions were avoided during focus group discussions.

In order to work with children or involve them in the study, several challenges had to be overcome. Permission had to be obtained from parents (as children are regarded as minors) and the Western Cape Education Department. Language was also a challenge, as many of the children were not always able to express themselves articulately. Understanding their perspectives posed a challenge. This was overcome by politely asking them to repeat their responses and by stating questions simply. Literacy problems were overcome by recording interviews instead of asking children to complete questionnaires. Generational issues also complicated the research process. The children regarded the researcher as an adult and, coupled with the sensitive nature of the research subject, it was initially difficult for them to easily open up. This was addressed by having ice breaker interactions prior to the interviews and focus group discussions.

Context of the children in the study

In order to fully appreciate the specificity of the South African context, a brief description of the contextual characteristics of each school is provided in Table 6.2 on page 66. Schools are not mentioned by name, to preserve confidentiality.

It is evident from the descriptions that there existed a strong variation in the socioeconomic status, parental background and racial demographics among the schools.

Table 6.2: Contextual characteristics of schools

School	Description
RP	The school is situated in a well-established suburb and historically catered for English-speaking white South Africans. Its demographic profile had since changed and it now consists of a diverse racial profile, including black, white and coloured children. All the parents at the school have professional careers, and school fees are paid regularly.
MP	The school is situated in a suburb that has numerous smaller suburban extensions. Houses in the school's neighbourhood are mostly two-bedroomed, similarly structured homes with a mainly coloured population. Twelve of the 39 respondents live in a black township, while the rest live in the immediate area of the school. Only one of the respondents' parents had a professional career.
SP	The school is situated in a relatively large area in which a range of religions and ways of life are evident. Religions include Christianity, Hinduism, Islam and others. The community comprises a diverse group as regards their economic status. The area has a variety of houses, ranging from economic homes and flats to semi-detached and free-standing luxury homes. From the learners' attire, it appeared that a large number of them in the class interviewed were poor.
LP	The school is situated in the southern suburbs of Cape Town, close to a sewerage site. The area is mainly occupied by black people. A large percentage of children do not have the necessary attire due to financial constraints. Out of the 42 respondents, only one of the children's fathers had a professional career. The rest worked as, for example, shoemakers, shop assistants, mine workers, maintenance workers, bakers and painters.
KP	The school is situated in a black residential area that consists of both a township and an informal settlement on the outskirts of Cape Town. Eight of the 34 respondents did not have direct access to running water, but only one respondent had no access to electricity. The school is situated in a poor area. The main entrance is unkempt and the school's office consists of only the bare essentials.

The descriptions given in Table 6.2 provide a context against which to interpret the study's findings.

Conceptual framework

Understandings of childhood have shifted from those that gave little recognition to children as having rights that are no different than those of adults. Much of this change has come about as a result of notions of children's identity expanding beyond essentialist biologism to include social conceptions that tend to view childhood more holistically (James et al, 1998). While sexuality among children in the past was perceived as a marginal phenomenon, holistic approaches to childhood have foregrounded children's sexuality as an important foundation of their identity construction.

In the age of modernity, theorists like Giddens (1987) offer a different perspective on sexuality as a more fluid feature of the self, namely as a major link connecting body, self, identity and social norms. This is further supported by Weeks (1986:15), who defines sexuality as a 'historical construction that brings together a host of different biological and mental possibilities – gender identity, bodily differences, reproductive capacities, needs, desires and fantasies'. McDermott (in Weeks, 1986) concurs with this definition when he argues that sexuality includes biological, social, cultural and psychological aspects that develop in a social context. The development of the sexual self, therefore, does not take place in isolation, but is context dependent. Dilley (1999:5) defines context as 'that which environs an object [and] suggests a range of synonyms such as environment, milieu, setting and background'; ie it comprises a generalised set of connections that shape the phenomena being investigated, and includes both the geographical and spatial (Dilley, 1999). Knowledge of context is pivotal in understanding sexual identity construction, and contexts within which sexual identity construction occurs are characterised by various factors, among them gender and HIV/AIDS.

In terms of the above, sexuality does not exist outside history, but is historically constructed. Each historical era, as Weeks (1986) suggests, heralds a new perspective on sexuality. A historical approach to sexuality in this work was useful in the sense that it exposed the power elements that determine the meanings people give to their lives in general and their sexual selves in particular. However, a historical approach to childhood and children's sexuality, as described by theorists such as Piaget, Freud, Kohlberg and Erickson (cited in Woodward, 2002), as well as Locke and Rousseau (see Burman, 1994), does not necessarily take into account the influence of the contexts in which the children grow up.

Woodward (2002) maintains that gender had been used as a concept that provided a focus for the social construction of femininity and masculinity, including hierarchical divisions between women and men based on social, political and economic practices and institutions. Gender was not viewed separately, but rather was conflated with sex. Feminist scholars such as Oakley (in Woodward, 2002) and Butler (1990) have attempted to disentangle gender from sex, with the former being a social construct. The differentiation is between sex as a biological and anatomical phenomenon and gender as the attributes that are associated with one or other sex in specific societies. To these scholars, therefore, gender can be viewed as a fluid variable that shifts and transforms in varied contexts and at varied times. The traditional construct of gender as a fixed variable continues to be challenged. In the post-modern era, the 'location' of gender seems to have shifted from a given or purely biological phenomenon to a construction, and gender is now regarded as a socially constructed phenomenon (Butler, 1990). Biological manifestations of maleness or femaleness are no guarantee that our sexual identities are formed in that way.

Epstein and Johnson (1998:152) explain that 'we … no longer "do" sexual acts, we are the acts we do, or, perhaps more accurately, the acts we identify with'. In order to develop an understanding of the ways in which sexuality is perceived in childhood, the context and historical period are important. Sexuality 'is always being produced, always changing and internally very diverse', bringing with it a 'discursive formation, a particular historical combination of discourses or discursive strategies with different histories' (Epstein & Johnson, 1998:16).

Sexual identity formation is strongly located in social constructions that are inscribed through social orders. Brah (in Weedon, 2000:129) maintains that 'questions of identity are intimately connected with those of experience … and social relations. [Sexual] identities are inscribed through experiences, subjectivity and social relations'. Experiences are determined by social relations and interaction with family, peers, media, class and religion (which form context), all of which play a major role in the determination of sexual identity formation. Epstein and Johnson (1998) argue that it is the family — in the axis of parent–child and not only the husband–wife axis — where an essential part of the social construction of sexuality takes place. Family not only influences children's sexuality, but also experiences and bears the weight of children's sexual issues.

This conceptual framework provides some interpretive tools for understanding the factors that shape sexual identity construction, and generally the manner in which children construct their sexual identities.

Main findings

Emerging from the data collected were the discursive spaces in which children made meaning of their sexual selves. These included the nature of the games they played and the extent to which these were gendered and sexualised, name calling, division of labour and the chores they performed in and out of school, and the influence of the media and religion on sexual identity.

Games children play

Games are one way in which children make sense of their everyday lives. They serve as a conduit for developing and understanding social relations within communities, between adults and children, and among children themselves. In some instances, games reflect community values and are thus a commentary on community beliefs and values, and offer a non-threatening space where children can act out what they experience in the communities in which they live. Games are also perceived as a space in which children make sense of their sexual selves, sometimes overtly and sometimes implicitly. Within this social practice, for the purpose of this study, children seemed to develop an understanding of what is and is not allowed, who is and is not allowed to speak, and the conditions under which these rules and restrictions operate. It is therefore through conditions of play that children learned the 'rules of the game' in their social environments.

Although the playing of games is intrinsic to childhood, there are factors that strongly influence the nature of the games they play. These factors include the different socioeconomic environments in which they find themselves, their gender and the sexual connotations evident in most games, as well as the formulation of rules within children's lore.

Socioeconomic environments

Different socioeconomic environments influenced the games children played. It appeared that self-invented games and traditional games that have been played for many generations were mainly played in poorer socioeconomic environments. Within such environments, it would seem that children were often more creative and innovative in the formulation or modification of games. In the focus group discussions, children from schools located in poorer socioeconomic environments (MP, SP, KP and LP) stated that they played games that included Abba ('horsy' or carrying each other on the back), which a girl at MP described as entailing 'getting on the boy's back'; 'poppiehuis' (doll's house); 'hide and seek'; and 'spin the bottle', all of which required limited physical resources.

Children at school RP, which is located in a rich neighbourhood, played some of the above games such as 'hide and seek', but mostly sports such as football, handball, and, most often, cricket.

Looking at the games played by children in the various schools, it is clear that the choice of games was to a great extent determined by the children's socioeconomic circumstances.

Gendered nature of games

Games played by these children were often gendered, and throughout the discussion of games, the impact of boy–girl relations was evident. The descriptions they gave implicitly and explicitly revealed the sexual connotations attached to the games that they played.

In school RP there were fixed games for boys and girls, while fluidity was evident in most of the other schools. However, when games included boys and girls, their sexual identities were invariably apparent, and, as a result, the games were markedly gendered. The 'expected' and 'accepted' behaviour and dispositions of boys and girls were often embedded in the rules or the nature of the games. Little questioning seemed to occur regarding either aspect. In most cases, the boys and girls played separately. Games such as football were perceived as games for boys, and in cases where girls played football matches with the boys, the latter still dominated. They took the lead and observations revealed that the girls seemingly toed the line in order to stay in the game. Girls also had to defend themselves for wanting to participate in a game dominated by the boys. Often, a boy who participated in the 'girls' games such as 'skipping rope' was regarded as a 'moffie' (a colloquial term used to refer to a male who displayed feminine characteristics).

Cross-gender games like 'hide and seek' and 'skipping rope' were also played. The girls, however, usually initiated these games. Boys were keen to play, but this usually started with an initial interaction in a teasing way between the girls and boys. At school SP, a particular cross-gender game was common that entailed running from pole to pole. The idea was that the girl would chase a boy and try to catch him between the poles. The boys would always catch the girls in a rather physical way, and girls responded in two different ways: either by angrily deterring the boys or laughingly gesticulating at them to 'control' themselves.

Sexual connotations and implications

Within the process of game playing and other observed activities, there appeared to be regular, if not persistent, allusions to sex. While it would be exaggerating to say that all the games that the children engaged in had sexual connotations, much of their interaction potentially had sexual implications. Some games resulted in interactions that could be described as being explicitly sexual in nature.

Several games were identified as having sexual connotations and implications. Such a game was 'spin the bottle'. Sharlene,[1] a pupil at SP, gave the following illustration: 'You spin

[1] For purposes of confidentiality, all the names used for schools and learners are fictitious.

the bottle and if that point faces you then they will dare you to do something between the girl and the boy .... The boy and the girl have to go in another room and kiss ... and take off your bra [brassiere] and all that ....' Simone added: 'When you take off your bra and show the boys, then the boys have to touch it [breasts]....' Another game with sexual connotations and implications was Abba. In describing some aspects of the game, Desiree, a girl from MP, said: 'They [boys] lie on us like they are attacking you or something ... it doesn't feel nice' (giggles and shakes head). 'Boys touch us everywhere.'

It seems emphasis in some of the games was no longer placed on the game itself, but on 'other' aspects that were often sexual in nature. These 'other' aspects were conveniently conducted as though they were integral aspects of the games. This occurred both consciously and unconsciously. The sexual connotations and aspects of the games were mainly determined by the space in which a particular game was played. It was observed that the games with distinct sexual connotations were played in spaces free from adult supervision. These 'private' spaces included the school playground and classroom and home environments, and these spaces conditioned the nature of the games.

Children therefore also created their own 'private' spaces, which were not merely confined to physical location. These spaces were set within a public setting where there were no adults present, thereby providing an ideal opportunity for them to play the games with sexual connotations and aspects. This was their way of making meaning of these particular spaces. Considering that the children chose spaces that were devoid of adults to engage in these games gives the impression that the sexual aspects were actually integral parts of the games. These games, it may be argued, were deliberately constructed and continuously reconstructed in such a manner that the children had the opportunity to 'explore' and express their sexualities.

It may be argued that some of the aspects of the games played by children discussed above (eg lying on top of each other, kissing, removing of brassieres and touching of breasts) coupled with the private spaces within which these games were played (especially in homes and even classrooms) may eventually lead to unprotected sex. These activities may initially happen as part of the 'game', but eventually develop into a habit.

Rules of the game

Within each game, rules played an essential role. Rules had both a literal and figurative application, since the 'game' not only referred to the children's lore, but also covered the wide spectrum of ways in which they determined their sexual identities. Rules were on the one hand literal, since they provided the actual boundaries or limitations set within each game to ensure the smooth flow of the game and the achievement of the ultimate outcome. On the other hand, however, these rules were figurative and enabled the sexual construction of specific patterns and behavioural nuances.

These rules were formulated in relation to the opposite gender and often appeared to be fluid. Games, as a social practice, therefore served as loci for the formation of these rules and patterns. The masculinity and femininity of the children were seemingly established within the essence of the social practices with which they gave substance to themselves.

Name calling and aggressive behaviour

During some of the games, it was evident that name calling and aggressive behaviour were often perpetuated. In this practice, the girls seemed to act as passive recipients, not only enduring bodily harm, but also slander and harsh utterances. The girls displayed minimal control over their choices. It was observed that at schools MP and LP, the girls were treated by the boys in a condescending manner. However, despite the manner in which these girls were treated, they subserviently tolerated the power display demonstrated by the boys. In doing so, they established certain rules regarding their femininity. Although they were aware of the implications, they tended to expose themselves to the continued victimisation dealt out by the boys. Desperation was evident and much tolerance was displayed. The boys' aggressive behaviour at schools KP, LP and MP, therefore, tended to shape the girls' feminine identity. This aggressive behaviour often went uncontested, thereby instilling the practice as a norm, and as being in the nature of boys.

Another form of 'aggressive' behaviour entailed what may be described as sexual harassment by the boys. It was reported that sometimes in the course of a game, the boys would sexually 'harass' the girls. Toby, a girl from school MP, explained:

> We have two friends — we play with them during interval. ... We play arm wrestling. Sometimes they take us ... hold us [and] sometimes their hands go there .... They smear us [and] they go with their hands to the lower body by the tummy. They are not supposed to do that to girls.

Amber, a girl from school MP, claimed the girls were complicit in their own harassment: 'The girls want to play with the boys. It's our own fault', she said. It appears that the aggressive behaviour of the boys and the girls' responses were patterned by a particular gendered script where boys (men) exercised power and girls (women) complied. Since the boys' aggressive behaviour went uncontested, it tended to get institutionalised or instilled as a norm, as evidenced by Sharlene from school SP, who believed that 'boys are like that'. In one of the schools, it emerged that some teachers played a role in encouraging aggressive behaviour by some boys. Amber from school MP narrated the following incidents involving a boy and how a teacher gave the impression that the boy's behaviour was acceptable: 'The boy in my class [will] touch you everywhere .... When we went on a field trip, he opened his zip. He lifted up a girl and started kissing her. The teacher was informed but nothing was done.' Even though both the boy's and the teacher's behaviour may have been an exception, by doing nothing even after he was informed of what had occurred, the teacher unfortunately conveyed the message that the boy's behaviour should be condoned. The teacher's response may also have reinforced the notion that 'boys are like that'. Such behaviour has implications for the way girls and even boys construct their sexual identities and negotiate relationships.

Chores

In addition to the games played and the name calling, the chores performed also served as an important means through which identity shaping occurred. A distinct impression of a division of labour was prevalent at schools MP, KP and LP. There was no chance of boys venturing onto the 'girls' territory.' The children alluded to the fact that the girls' physical strength and biological makeup were designed to enable them to perform particular chores, and it was an accepted norm that certain duties were assigned strictly according to specific genders. At schools SP and RP, however, although the children had specific duties to perform, they were willing to share responsibilities and were not bound to a fixed division of labour.

An interesting revelation was the responses that children gave relating to their parents' participation in chores. Beverly, a pupil at school MP, described her father's role thus: 'My father is the head of the house. He is the boss of the house. Payments are his responsibilities.' Carlin, also a pupil at school MP, described her mother's role thus: 'She must be there. She buys food, clothing ... she does the work.' The parents, it seemed, set the framework for the manner in which chores and activities were done at home.

Overall, gender differences were revealed in the chores that the children were involved in. Out of the dominant discourse of heterosexuality emerged the discursive formation of dichotomised gender roles. Biological inscription, which included physical strength, seemed to be the determining factor. The findings demonstrated how children constructed their sexual identities by either resisting or reproducing the dichotomised gender roles offered by society.

Media and sexual identity

It has already been pointed out that many influences served as loci for the construction of sexual identity for children. It was evident that television, sibling and parental influences, and religion contributed immensely to sexuality construction in children. Children from MP, KP and RP expressed that the television specifically enabled them to pursue or constrained them from pursuing certain activities that had a direct impact on the manner in which their sexual identities were constructed. The learners acknowledged that the temptation to imitate whatever they saw on television was significant. Toby, a learner from school MP, stated: 'Children want to do it [imitate what they watch on television]. The boys talk about *Emmanuelle* [a semi-pornographic movie on a local television channel].' Kaylene from school KP added: 'TV can show you things you are not supposed to do and it can change you. It is not good to watch TV with lots of sex. You can dream about those things.'

The influence of the media, as intimated by Toby, may have a snowball effect. By discussing the sexual programmes at school, it is unlikely that those who do not watch the programmes will not be influenced. Through some of the games discussed earlier, coupled with peer pressure, the learners could be tempted to 'enact' certain television scenes with a sexual orientation. Thus, exposing children to 'sex', whether via discussion or drama, played an influential role in the way in which they perceived themselves and demonstrated their sexual identities. If left unaddressed by parents and teachers, among others, whatever children observed on television was more likely to be interpreted as fashionable and desirable.

Transcending the biological boundaries

Not all children adhered to the normative discourse or sets of practices available to them. At school MP, an unexpected finding emerged. After a discussion on chores, one participant seemed to be shaping her sexuality by transcending the biological boundaries. She was female, but her disposition, attitude and utterances illustrated a defiance of her 'existing gender'. She enjoyed playing with the boys, and the topics of her conversations were orientated around her male friends' interests. The learner, Toby, was very close to her brother. She was called a tom-boy and had interests in wrestling and scary movies, and enjoyed the company of boys. She said of herself: 'I don't like "girlie" stuff. I play wrestling, soccer and boys' stuff.' These factors have seemingly shaped her sexual identity, one that challenges essentialised and gendered sexual identities.

Toby's 'acquired' sexual identity was frowned upon by the other learners, who mobilised religious arguments as their basis for contesting her sexual identity. This identity was seen as an anomaly and was questioned in terms of 'God's creation plan'. Specific statements were made that enhanced the notion that everyone was created either male or female and that this biological state was not to be questioned. For instance, Kurt from school MP said: 'Jesus said you are the girl [and] you are not going to change.' Toby was, however, adamant in displaying her inward convictions regarding her sexual identity, even though this attitude, according to her peers, was in total contradiction to Christian beliefs. She displayed a growing desire to medically undergo a sex change. This response further elicited discussion of Christian religious beliefs. Her response, in particular, highlighted religion as a strong basis for the way in which most of her peers perceived their masculinity and femininity.

Discussion

The various factors shaping children's sexual identity construction that have been discussed above suggest that children seemingly construct their sexual identities through different influences within complex discursive spaces. Although certain influences seem to be stronger than others, ultimately, it should be understood that several influences impact on the children simultaneously and, in some cases, reinforce one another. Generally, these influences, embedded in predominantly heterosexual discourses, seem to perpetuate a distinct behavioural trend that masculinises and feminises children's sexual identities in particular ways that work to reinscribe the dominant discourse and its concomitant social practices.

The games children play influence the construction of their sexual identities. As shown in the foregoing discussion, through games or interactive play, gender identities are produced, reproduced and regulated. Through these social practices, girls learn about 'girlishness' and boys about 'boyishness'. These social practices therefore serve as loci for the formation of rules and patterns. Dispositions become rule-constructing opportunities that directly impact on children's masculinity and femininity. The rules of the games have both a literal and figurative application, since these 'games' not only refer to the children's lore, but also covers the wider spectrum of sexual identity construction.

Given the context of HIV/AIDS in which children live, the processes through which they construct their sexual identities are crucial. Of particular concern is the sexual nature of some of the games played and the possibility of such games leading to risky sexual behaviour. But of more significance is the apparent acceptance of male hegemony and female submission as normal and accepted practice. The hegemonic behaviour and dispositions of boys vis-à-vis the 'performances' by girls could encourage sexual harassment of girls by boys and also inhibit the negotiation of safe sexual relationships.

Conclusion

It is clear from the foregoing discussion that social worlds, as contexts, stimulate and ultimately mould personalities and sexual identity formations (Walker, Reid & Cornell, 2004). These social worlds appear to be essential context-forming factors that contribute to the development of predispositions, hereby creating the location that develops the construction of sexual identity (Bourdieu, 1993). The routine involvement that children have in their social worlds enables them to acquire tendencies to act and view issues in particular ways.

In the quest to establish some ways in which children construct their sexual identities, this chapter has shown the following:

- Children construct their sexual identities within a context-dependent and situation-specific environment. Socioeconomic factors and historical background in particular play a major role in the shaping of their sexuality.
- The activities children occupy themselves with, such as games, chores and entertainment, are all social practices in which they sexually position themselves in particular ways. Involvement in these activities enhances the shaping of masculinity and femininity. It is evident that children are actively engaged in establishing the 'rules of the game' while being immersed in their daily activities. These formulated rules serve as a framework that determines their dispositions, resulting in them masculinising or feminising their behaviour.
- Many institutions and agents directly influence the ways in which children are shaped sexually. Parents and siblings, through interaction, communication and modelling behaviour, prescribe the prerequisites and formulation of sexual identity construction, hereby enhancing the shaping process. In addition to this, the visual and auditory strengths of the media contribute to the way in which sexual constructions occur.
- The dominant discourse of heterosexuality can be challenged. One learner, the 'anomaly', constructed her sexual identity by transcending the boundaries of her biological gender. The confines of the physical have not prevented her from exploring and questioning her femaleness and partially replacing these nuances with masculine tendencies. This emphasises the duality of gender construction, rather than seeing it as a biological manifestation.

Overall, the findings of the study have revealed that sexuality in relation to children cannot be viewed as a separate entity, but as an integrated process to which children dynamically contribute as they continually construct and deconstruct their sexual developmental experience.

Chapter 7

Mamatsoso Matsoso-Makhate
with Gerald Wangenge-Ouma
University of Cape Town

Performing Masculine and Feminine Identities: Sexuality and Identity Construction among Youth in the Context of HIV/AIDS

Introduction

Young people, especially adolescents, are considered to be among the most susceptible to HIV infection. In South Africa, as in many countries throughout the world, high incidence of HIV/AIDS infection is found among the youth. It is estimated that 961 000 South African youth between the ages of 15–24 were living with HIV/AIDS in 2004 (Dorrington et al, 2004). Of the nine provinces of South Africa, KwaZulu-Natal was estimated as having the highest HIV/AIDS prevalence rate of 19.7% among youth aged 15–24 in 2002. While the prevalence rates in the Western Cape (3.3%) remain low, the province is said to show the fastest escalation of infections.

A large part of the risk of HIV infection facing adolescents concerns the challenge they face in dealing with in terms of coping with changes in their bodies and their feelings. This challenge involves a search for identity and the need to relate to others in an intimate way. Adolescence is a period typified by feelings of pleasure, desire and becoming a well-rounded person (Coleman & Roker, 1998). According to DiClemente (1992), adolescence is a period during which many young people will initiate sexual and drug-related risk behaviour that increases the probability of HIV infection.

The vulnerability of young people to HIV infection is complex. It arises out of the fact that most have not yet selected their life partners and are likely to change sexual partners often (Skinner, 2000). Some young people are also at risk of HIV/AIDS infection because of factors such as substance use (abuse) and other socioeconomic factors such as poverty, which may lead to early engagement in sexual activities in return for money or other favours (UNAIDS, 2000; Wangenge-Ouma, 2007). Risk taking is also influenced by the sociocultural context in which youth learn the norms of society, what society expects of them and where they learn about who they are sexually. Through social interactions, youth learn culturally informed norms that influence their sexuality and determine their sexual behaviours (LeClerc-Madlala, 2001).

Several studies have been carried out on youth and HIV/AIDS. These studies have focused on various aspects, among others, knowledge, attitudes and perceptions regarding HIV/AIDS (Van Wijk, 1994; Sally, 1990; Levine & Ross, 2002; Makhate, 2002); the relationship between knowledge of and attitudes towards HIV/AIDS and sexual behaviours and decision making (Kelly et al, 2002); decision making and sexual risk taking

(Varga, 1997; Lugoe & Klepp, 1996; Skinner, 2001); and the link between knowledge of HIV/AIDS and behaviour, with a focus on why there are still high HIV infection rates among youth despite their perceived knowledge of how the disease is transmitted and how to protect themselves (LeClerc-Madlala, 2002a; Wangenge-Ouma, 2007). These studies have produced various results. For example, the studies by Levine and Ross (2002), Makhate (2002) and Wangenge-Ouma (2007) show that despite youth's engagement in (risky) sexual activities, they did not regard themselves as an at-risk group. For them, AIDS was a disease for 'other' people, such as promiscuous men and women, prostitutes, drug addicts and the poor.

Studies by, among others, Varga (1997), Lugoe and Klepp (1996) and Skinner (2001) focusing on decision making and sexual risk taking show that young people engage in risky sexual behaviours and that generally there is inequality in sexual decision making, where it seems boys are in control. The studies also report cases where girls engage in sex just to please their sexual partners. LeClerc-Madlala's (2002a) and Wangenge-Ouma's (2007) studies, which examine the relationship among the youth, HIV/AIDS and the importance of understanding sexual cultures and contexts, report cases of young women engaging in quasi-consensual survival sex, whereby they understood sex as a resource that could be drawn upon for material or economic advantage, for example, in securing jobs; getting gifts such as clothes; or acquiring basic needs such as school fees, food and rent.

A few studies have examined youth sexual identity construction and ways in which this may influence youth's sexual decision making, their negotiation of safe sex and their response to HIV/AIDS. One such study is that by Reddy (2003), which looked at troubling sexualities and sexual identity construction in the context of HIV/AIDS among students in a secondary school in KwaZulu-Natal. She found that the students were making sense of their sexual selves under socially given conditions that included gendered structures of power and social relations. For example, 'soft' emotions were associated with girls and 'aggressive' ones with boys (Reddy, 2003:175). The study on which this chapter is based sought to contribute to this emerging body of knowledge. It investigated how adolescents constructed their sexual identities in the context of HIV/AIDS, how they viewed themselves as sexual beings, and how they negotiated and presented themselves in relationships. The study also looked at how adolescents performed their femininity and masculinity in the construction of their sexual identities and how this led to unequal power relations and agency within their relationships. This chapter's main focus is the construction of adolescents' sexual identities in the context of HIV/AIDS.

Methodology

As mentioned above, the main objective of the study was to find out how adolescents construct their sexual identities in the context of HIV/AIDS. The study's focus was on what and how social practices inform and shape youth's construction of their sexual identities and how youth conceive of their sexuality. To achieve the study's objectives, a qualitative research approach was utilised.

Sampling

Pseudonyms were used for both schools and respondents to ensure confidentiality. The study was conducted in four coeducational and purposively sampled secondary schools in Western Cape Province, South Africa. These schools, namely Radford, Heritage, Zingisani and De Hoop were selected to ensure the inclusion of respondents from different socioeconomic backgrounds, races and religious affiliations.

Radford is a predominantly white school, and most of the learners come from middle-class families. Heritage is a predominantly coloured school, with varying numbers of Muslim and Christian learners. The school is located in an area comprising both middle-class and working-class families. Zingisani is located in a black township characterised by high unemployment and poverty. It is a small school and all the learners and the majority of the teachers are Xhosa speaking. De Hoop Secondary School is located in a predominantly coloured Afrikaans-speaking working-class community containing large numbers of unemployed people. Most of the learners in the school come from single-parent families or are living with their grandparents.

In each of the four schools, grade 9 learners aged 14–18 years were selected. Grade 9 learners were selected because they were at the adolescent stage and were experiencing both physical and emotional changes. The assumption was that they were also at an age where they were thinking about, exploring or engaging in some form of sexual activity. This was an important factor, since the study focused on sexual identity construction.

Regarding the sampling of the participants in the study, it was initially intended that since each school had several grade 9 streams, participants would be selected from each stream. This was not possible, as the schools' management argued that such an approach would disrupt the smooth running of classes. In each school, therefore, the management identified one grade 9 class to be involved in the study. No specific criterion was provided for the selection of these classes, though in two schools that had Afrikaans- and English-medium classes, the English-medium class was selected. The number of learners in each of the selected classes ranged between 20 and 40.

The selection of the learner sample occurred in phases and varied from the use of entire classes for the completion of a questionnaire to the selection of a few individuals for focus group discussions and individual interviews. Overall, the study had a questionnaire sample of 124 learners, a focus group sample of 32 learners and an individual interview sample of 16 learners. Several learners were included in all three samples. As already alluded to above, data was collected using a questionnaire, focus group discussions and interviews. Observations were also conducted.

Ethical considerations

Understanding sexual identity involves dealing with issues relating to sexual behaviours, which are often considered as secret, intimate, sometimes taboo and often very personal. The sensitivity of the topic is usually due to the way in which most societies' 'areas of social life concerned with sexual … matters remain shielded from the eyes of non-intimates' (Claire & Lee, 1993:6).

Apart from the sensitive nature of the topic, the study also dealt with adolescents between the ages of 14–18 years. As a result, explicit questions could not be asked, and attention had to be paid to the places where the interviews were being conducted, as well as the nature of the questions asked. Also, community and school viewpoints on sex and sexuality were respected.

Before the study was conducted, consent was obtained from the Department of Education, the four schools and the learners' parents. Seeking parental consent was necessary, since the learners were below the age of 18 (it is a mandatory requirement that studies involving children under the age of 18 seek the consent of the children's parents) and the subject being studied was also sensitive. The learners were also briefed about the study and were informed that participation was voluntary and that they were free to discontinue their participation at any time.

Conceptual framework

It is acknowledged that adolescent years are characterised by the search for identity. It is a period when people begin to ask questions related to 'Who am I?' (Erikson, 1968) and attempt to make sense of their place within society. It is therefore a time when collective/social identities, personal identities and sexual identities are all brought into question (Erikson, 1968).

Understanding adolescent identity means examining constructions of identity, and this in turn means examining how society works (Hall & Du Gay, 1996). It further means paying particular attention to the relations between social agents themselves and the nexus between social agents and institutions that shape and are shaped by the social actors (Hall & Du Gay, 1996). Societies shape how we make sense of our personal and collective identities and the ways in which we experience our lives. Understanding adolescent development therefore needs to take into account how identity is constructed and the context in which it is constructed.

Identities are points of temporary attachment to the subject position, which discursive practices construct for us (Hall & Du Gay, 1996:6); ie we cannot talk of personal identity without referring to the society within which we construct this identity. Skinner (in Breakwell, 1992) suggests that social identity is personal identity and personal identity is social identity, meaning that they coexist and intermix.

Identities are complex, as they are not 'an already accomplished fact' that one associates with oneself, but 'are the names we give to the different ways we are positioned by and position ourselves within the narratives of the past' (Hall, 1990:23). Hall (1990) suggests that identity construction is influenced by the sociocultural practices within the contexts in which we find ourselves. He further argues that identities are invented through attempts to represent them. In addition, Hall (1990) maintains that identity is a production that is never complete, always in process, and constituted within, not outside, representation. Identities therefore keep on changing and depend on the social settings in which we are positioned and position ourselves (Hall, 1990). Hall further adds that we act and say things from a position in context, and that we speak from a particular place and time, and from a history and a culture that are specific.

Hogg and Abrams (1988) argue that social identity is qualitatively different from individual identity, and that the group is somehow contained in the mind of the individual group member. In this sense, individual behaviour is influenced by as much as it influences group behaviour (Hogg & Abrams, 1988). Social identity is a result of the individual's knowledge that he/she belongs to certain social groups, together with some emotional and value significant to the individual or the group members (Tajfel in Hogg & Abrams, 1988:7).

Bourdieu (1976) adds that social identity is a sense of the position one occupies in a social space and acknowledges that societies, like other institutions, have dominant discourses and that power relations exist within which people are positioned and position themselves. This implies that in societies, those groups that possess power and weight have a social position that makes it possible for them to create a dominant hegemonic culture (Bourdieu, 1976). Societies shape individuals and at the same time depend entirely upon the actions and dispositions of individuals for their existence. This means that actors do not simply follow rules, but bend them and work around them so as to maximise their own best advantage, and, in the long run, some of these rules change (Crossley, 2001). Bourdieu (1976) adds that identity construction depends on the societies and institutions in which we find ourselves, as what exists as reality for the individual is to a great degree determined by what is socially acceptable. For Bourdieu, schools, for example, provide those who have been subjected directly or indirectly to their influence with general dispositions that generate particular patterns that can be applied in different areas of thought and action. Bourdieu (1976) calls this 'cultural habitus'.

Regarding the project to create a sense of self, Giddens (1991) suggests that the 'self' as 'me' can only be understood when the 'I' is understood in relation to the discourse of the 'other'. 'Self' is perceived as both the object and subject due to the self-reflective nature of human beings, as there is a 'me' for the 'I' to reflect upon, and it is assumed that the 'I' is a cognitive structure in the form of a self-concept (Hogg & Abrams, 1988:24). In this case, Hogg and Abrams (1988) maintain that the 'I' is responsible for constructing the 'me'. Identity construction is therefore a discovery and affirmation of the innate essence that determines what 'I am', while it is also argued that it is created from available social roles. What 'I am' is therefore dependent on social feedback from others (Hogg & Abrams, 1988).

Adolescence as a distinct identity has been conceptualised in various ways. Theories of human development (Piaget in Muuss, 1988; Erikson, 1968; Kohlberg in Muuss 1988) view adolescence as a stage of human development in which people behave in a particular and predictable way. The main limitation of human development theories is that they universalise children's development and do not take into account individual differences and the contexts in which identity is constituted. They therefore ignore the complexity and multiple factors that inform and shape human development in the context in which this development occurs. Thus, human development theories do not take into consideration the individual agent and the social context in which the agent makes meaning of his/her environment.

Jessor (1998), Allen-Meares and Shapiro (1989), and Crockett and Crouter (1995), among others, provide very useful and holistic perspectives on adolescence. Jessor (1998) argues that society plays a role in shaping who we are and how we behave, and gives meaning to our experiences. Thus, changes occurring during adolescence are defined by an individual's social context and by the roles and expectations for behaviour, based on an individual's identification with or membership in a social group. Identification here means the degree of recognition of sameness to or connectedness with social identity. The social groups one identifies with may, for example, be social classes, peer groups, parental and school influences, and images in the media (Allen-Meares & Shapiro, 1989).

Crockett and Crouter (1995) also posit that the pathways taken by adolescents depend on the environment in which they are developing. This may include families, peers and the local neighbourhood. These people/institutions, they argue, shape the actual opportunities available for adolescents, as well as risks to which they are exposed.

Adolescence is also viewed as a period characterised by an upsurge of sexual drives, the development of sexual values and the initiation of sexual behaviours (Jessor, 1998). These include physical, cognitive and emotional aspects, all of which play a role in the decision-making process of adolescents. Adolescent development, it would seem, has to be understood in a much more holistic way. This involves understanding the interrelationship among physical, cognitive and emotional development, as well as understanding that these operate within a particular context. Understanding adolescent development as embedded in contexts is important in examining why youth may engage in behaviours that put them at risk of being infected with HIV.

The foregoing conceptual framework provides an interpretive lense through which the construction of sexual identities by the adolescent learners in the study is understood. The point is emphasised that the construction of sexual identities, like other identities, is a product of a range of factors, key among them being the context in which the individual is located. This context includes social actors, structures, and social and cultural practices to which actors contribute and through which people give meaning to their collective and personal identities. The discussion that follows, an exploration of how adolescent learners construct their sexual identities, is guided by this conceptual framework. The main argument in the discussion is that adolescent learners construct their sexual identities through understanding their respective gendered roles in initiating, negotiating and managing relationships.

Main findings

What follows reveals that sexual identity construction among youth occurs largely through decisions about and subsequent actions shaping, in particular, heterosexual relationships. Gendered role identifications were prominent, making relationship decision making an important discursive space for sexual identity construction.

Initiating relationships: Who pursues and who is pursued?

The study's results revealed two main features about how sexual identities are understood in the process of initiating relationships. The first relates to an awareness of expected roles and how this awareness leads to the second aspect, the 'performance' of an expected role. Within the latter, evidence emerged of how practices are sometimes subverted, particularly by females.

Regarding the first aspect, the responses in the study revealed that in initiating relationships, the dominant trend was that boys are 'pursuers' while girls are the 'pursued'.

All the 32 learners in the focus group discussions (FGDs), irrespective of gender and racial group, maintained that it was the male's role to initiate relationships or to go out and seek a partner. Dilikhaya, an older and mature boy among those interviewed in Zingisani, stated: 'The boy *has* [his emphasis] to approach the girl, not the girl.' Allen, a white boy from Radford, also held similar views as the above. He stated: 'It's the guy that approaches the girl usually. I don't know if its dominance or whatever, but the guy usually has … to do it in a sense.'

Interestingly, all girls, irrespective of their race or geographic location, were 'aware' that initiating and negotiating relationships fell within the 'expected' role of boys. Laura, a white girl from Radford, captured a common view when she stated: 'I don't really go straight up to a guy and tell him I like him or something like that ... I still prefer them to come to me.' While it was a common trend among this group of learners that boys had to initiate relationships, there were boys and girls who felt that girls could also initiate relationships. While there may be an acceptance of a different role for girls, boys still controlled the process, since it was they who decided whether or not to pursue a relationship once approached by a girl.

The girls from Radford seemed comfortable with the view that boys pursue and they (the girls) are the pursued. Interestingly, the coloured and black girls voiced differing opinions. Charne, from Heritage, said she would approach a boy if she liked him: 'If I like a boy and he doesn't come to me, then I go to him.' Interestingly, though, the same girls who felt they could initiate relationships had never actually done so. When asked why, the black girls from Zingisani said they feared disappointment and being labelled as loose. Nosizo said: 'Girls are scared to talk to boys because they will say, *"umtwana ke sfebe"* [that girl is a whore].' Charmaine, a coloured girl from Heritage, concurred with this view. Her reluctance to initiate a relationship emanated from fear of rejection. This, she suggested, would create feelings associated with a low sense of self-worth.

Social networks and initiating practices

An awareness of the 'expected' roles for males and females seemed to produce intricate ways in which girls in particular produced practices that on the surface could be perceived as passive, but, when examined, were actually active. Generally, all the girls understood that they could not approach a boy directly, because that was not 'expected' of them. What emerged, therefore, was the use of a series of networks that included the use of friends, 'bumping into each other', and what was termed 'the look'. These practices, it would seem, ensured that dominant roles were maintained and that these girls appeared as being 'pursued' and passive.

The girls from Heritage and Radford argued that friends played a role in initiating and negotiating relationships. They suggested that in cases where they liked a boy, they often felt they could not approach him directly. Instead, they told a friend, who would then tell the boy so that he could pursue the girl. The girl, on the other hand, would pretend that she was being pursued.

Interestingly, the boys from the four schools did not mention using friends to initiate relationships, but they seemed to be aware of the way in which these girl networks operated and responded to them in unquestioning ways. The use of friends, it would seem, was a means by which girls could assert themselves and make choices about who they wanted to be in a relationship with, thereby not accepting it as solely the prerogative of the boys. Interestingly, though, it was done in a way that made boys assume control of whatever choice they made.

Choice of partners and sexual identity

As has already been discussed above, within this cohort of respondents, the choice of partners seemed to be influenced by the different expected masculine and feminine roles. Through their choice of partners, the adolescents seemed to be making sense of their sexual identities. In the main, they seemed to idealise what for them was feminine or masculine. This included a particular body image and personality, as well as specific dress codes. How choices were made, though, was interesting. In general, choice for boys seemed to be based on girls' personality. For some, honesty was also a consideration, but looks seemed to be the most important consideration. All the four boys from Zingisani not only considered looks as important, but also the girls' body size. Andile stated: 'She should not be big ... not fat, not thin. Just in the middle. She has to be beautiful.' For girls, values of honesty and trust took precedence. There were, however, individual differences in the emphasis on certain characteristics that varied across race and geographic location.

For girls, though, while there were differences in the characteristic features of an ideal partner, there seemed to be a general agreement that ideal partners had to be honest and trustworthy. So, while looks and personality were dominant factors in considering choice of partners, many girls said that for the most part, this was not the main consideration. Emphasis on different features varied across race and geographic location. The four girls at Radford emphasised personality and intelligence. Two girls from Zingisani stressed that they liked boys who were trustworthy and who had similar interests to them. The four girls from De Hoop seemed to place confidence in looks and the ability to care. They maintained that they would like someone who was handsome, loved them and could take care of them.

While contextually there were differences among this cohort, they commonly placed emphasis on looks, personality, values such as honesty and trust, and intelligence. It would seem that those from the more affluent environments placed emphasis on intelligence, whereas those from poorer environments emphasised looks and personality. It would also seem, though, that while boys and girls were in general agreement on some common features, unlike the boys, girls considered age and conceptions of boys as important identifying features in making a choice.

Age was an important consideration for 14 of the 16 girls in the FGDs. They all argued that they wanted to be in relationships with older boys. Interestingly, reasons for the need of an age difference seemed to differ by race and geographic location. The consensus among the four girls from Zingisani was that older boys were more experienced in relationships, and girls could therefore learn from them. Nosizo stated: 'I like older boys; they teach you, like my boyfriend last year he said I should kiss him and I didn't know and he said just kiss me I will show you.' Among the girls at De Hoop, older partners were expected to offer security and support. Shirley implied this when she stated: 'If he is younger than you [then] you have to be like his mother or something, you have to look after him.' Thus, it seems girls began to understand themselves as the weaker gender compared to their male partners. Rita added: 'He has to take care of me.'

Older partners were also given preference by the girls at Heritage, but the reasons differed from those offered above. For them, boys their age or younger were less mature and often childish. Charne stated: 'Boys our age are childish; if you say you want to spend time with them, they will say, "not now, I'm going to watch Superman"' (laughter). The preference for older boys and the reasons given seem to suggest that the girls considered the boys' maturation as being slower than theirs.

Control, restrictions and sexual identity

Relationships are not neutral places, but rather spaces in which power relations are manifested in gendered ways. Very often, boys had more control in relationships. The expectation that boys should initiate relationships implicitly ascribed to boys some privilege in terms of the power balance in the relationship. Their performance of this role seemed to encourage the notion that the relationship was the product of their (the boys') efforts. The power differentials in relationships had an influence on the way in which boys and girls began to understand their sexual identities.

Due to the recognisable power relations, some girls felt that being in a relationship restricted their freedom. However, responses differed across gender and geographic location. One girl from Radford and another from Heritage felt that they did not want to be in relationships at their age, for reasons associated with control. Carol from Radford stated:

> I don't have a boyfriend now, I prefer to stay free, it's nicer. It's just [that] if you want to do something you can just go ahead and do it. Boys can [be] very possessive. I don't want to be stuck with this because at this time in my life I like going around saying hi, how's it, what's your name, what are you doing, you know.

Carol's family background may also have influenced the decision. Her parents were divorced and she did not believe that relationships could last. She stated: 'I'm scared that what happened with my parents, [who] must have loved each other, [may also] happen to me. Too much stress!' (laughs).

Charne from Heritage expressed the same sentiment when she added that having a boyfriend meant: 'You did not have to love other people and the boyfriend has to know where you are every time.' For this reason, she felt she was 'still too young to think about love and … I'm just going out with that boy to have fun to enjoy my young life. I like a lot of guys; I can't stick to one … that's why I would rather joll.' These two girls felt they did not want to be in relationships, because it would limit their freedom.

While the girls from Heritage and Radford found relationships restrictive, the girls in De Hoop and Zingisani seemed to take for granted that relationships took place in this manner. For example, Thobeka's relationship seemed to be controlled by her boyfriend, because they could only see each other when he requested. She was satisfied with the arrangement, because, as she argued, this spared her from being hurt. She stated: 'I wait for him to call me and ask me to come over. I don't want to come to his place and maybe find him with another girl. I can be frustrated.'

Unlike the girls, where restriction seemed to be associated with power and control, and thus assumed heterosexual positions of masculinity and femininity, restriction for boys was associated with freedom to date more than one girl. Shane, a coloured boy from Heritage, summed it up in this way: 'We [himself and a former girlfriend] agreed we would still be friends because you can't see the same person the whole of your life and so on.'

Discussion

As the foregoing data shows, heterosexuality seemed to frame the ways in which boys and girls made sense of their expected roles and how they positioned and were positioned within the various phases of initiating, negotiating and embarking on the actual relationship. While the nature of this engagement was embedded within an understanding of the expected feminine and masculine roles, what the data revealed was a nuanced series of performances that 'played' into these perceived roles and on the surface subscribed to the 'expected'. The students seemed to perform their gendered roles, where males were perceived as 'initiators' and females as the 'pursued', even in circumstances that allowed for subversion of such roles. A study by Harrison et al (2001) also demonstrates that gender roles drove the respondents' experiences of their sexuality, where boys were expected to determine the nature of the relationships they had with girls. This may imply that girls are passive in the initiating and negotiating of their relationships, while boys are active. However, the discussion suggests that dichotomising feminine and masculine roles into distinct categories of 'the pursuer' and 'the pursued' obscures the complex ways in which the discourse is, on the one hand, maintained and, on the other, subverted.

A striking feature in the study's findings was how girls in particular understood those roles as a 'performance', while boys, on the other hand, just knew and accepted that it was always so. Girls were active in both maintaining and subverting the discourse where, for example, by using networks in initiating relationships, they underplayed the expectation that boys were the ones who would have an interest in girls and then pursue them. However, in their use of networks, girls still accorded boys the opportunity of performing the role of initiator, because after they had shown their interest in the boys, the latter were still the ones making the decision of whether or not to pursue the girl.

In playing into these roles, girls subscribed and complied with predetermined sets of hierarchical power relations, thereby positioning the boys higher and thus reducing the girls' power of negotiation within a relationship. These findings coincide with Varga's (1997) study, where he found that males were often in control and girls adhered to their partners' demands. While his study related particularly to the Zulu culture, where, in power relations, women were taught to be submissive, while men were supposed to be strong and assertive, the present study revealed a dominance of this pattern irrespective of race, ethnicity or geographic location. Even though girls at the four schools illustrated contrasting responses to the issue of power and control within relationships, the dominant pattern was still one of male control and female surrender. While girls from Radford and Heritage manifested some level of control, they had not actualised this in current relationships. At De Hoop and Zingisani, some girls accepted this ultimate control by the boys, taking for granted that heterosexual relationships operated in this way.

The power relations within relationships may also be a result of the age difference within relationships, as girls often preferred older boys. This was also suggested in Harrison et al (2001), where age was a determining factor in relationships. The reasons for this preference for older boys varied among the girls in this study. Unlike in Harrison et al's (2001) study, where older men were preferred because they could offer money and other material goods, the girls in the present study preferred older boys because, apparently, they could offer the time to be with their girlfriends. Older boys were also considered a form of security, because, apparently, they could 'take care' of their girlfriends and were also supposedly experienced in relationships. Boys their age or younger, on the other hand, were considered immature or childish and 'inexperienced' in relationships. This age difference may be a contributing factor that helps explain why girls are sometimes rendered powerless within relationships. This may also be the reason why girls usually have difficulty in negotiating safe sex or delaying sex with their partners.

What emerges is a picture of youth constructing sexual identities from predominantly heterosexual positions. Many taken-for-granted assumptions are upheld within these sexual constructions. Women are expected to be aesthetically appealing and complacent, while men are supposedly the caretakers, controllers of relationships and intelligent. What emerges, therefore, is a portrait of, particularly, girls unquestioningly complying in maintaining the status quo of male privilege.

Although adolescents also employ their agency in constructing their sexual identities, from the discussion, it appears that the environment in which they are located (expected patterns of behaviour) has the greater influence on the sexual identities that they assume. There is a greater tendency to 'fit in' and behave in expected ways. As already pointed out, this has implications in the context of HIV/AIDS. It is not unlikely, therefore, that adolescents may engage in risky sexual behaviour as they perform their 'expected' roles.

The HIV/AIDS context that adolescents live in requires that they develop sexual identities that do not put them at risk of infection. This will require that adolescents employ their agency in a more critical way when constructing their sexual identities rather than merely performing their gendered roles. Developing 'safe' sexual identities may require that some gendered roles, eg submissiveness among women and having multiple sexual partners among men, be subverted.

Conclusion

The foregoing discussion revealed that masculinities and femininities as distinct identities are constantly created, adapted and contested in everyday interactions (Reddy, 2003). As shown in the discussion, established masculinities and femininities can be seen as 'imitative text' (Butler, 1990). The boys and girls in this study demonstrated the complexities involved in the construction of their sexual identities through situated gendered performances. Overall, the learners seemed to understand what was expected of them and then performed the expected feminine and masculine roles.

This awareness of expected roles led to various performances where, on the one hand, the learners played into the expected roles, such as the pursuer and the pursued. On the other hand, an understanding of these roles as performances led to girls subverting them in ways that included, for example, making use of friends in initiating relationships. Relationships seemed to be one of the most important discursive spaces where the learners in this study made sense of their sexual selves. Through involvement in initiating, negotiating and participating in actual relationships, they seemed to produce particular sexual identities that were premised on heterosexual hierarchies. Girls, it seems, reinscribed identities of sexual powerlessness by, among other things, using social networks and choosing older boys. Boys, on the other hand, seemed to accept roles unquestioningly and assumed that particular roles were expected of them.

The construction of sexual identities by performing 'expected' gendered roles, especially for girls, could have far-reaching implications, especially in the context of HIV/AIDS. As indicated in the discussion, the expected gendered roles, and other factors such as age difference, tilted power relations in favour of boys. Consequently, this could undermine girls' exercise of agency in making choices regarding, for example, safe sex and condom use.

Chapter 8

Julia Kate Nupen
with Gerald Wangenge-Ouma
University of Cape Town

Grade 10 Learners' Conceptions of Risk of HIV Infection in Four Secondary Schools in the Western Cape

Introduction

This chapter focuses on young people's perceptions and understandings of risk in the context of HIV/AIDS. The chapter is extracted from a study that attempted to answer the following question: What are grade 10 learners' conceptions of risk in four secondary schools in the Western Cape and how do these conceptions influence relationship choice making in the context of HIV/AIDS?

The study was motivated by the existing gap between young people's knowledge of HIV/AIDS and their conceptions of risk of infection. For example, research conducted by Netswera (2002) and Simbayi et al (2005) found that despite having high levels of knowledge about HIV/AIDS, youth's attitudes and behaviour generally seemed unchanged. They also did not seem fearful of contracting the disease and practised high-risk behaviour.

HIV/AIDS-related deaths among South African youth aged 10–24 have increased from 22 636 in 1997 to 38 054 in 2004 (AVERT, 2007). This indicates a 68% increase in HIV/AIDS-related deaths for this age category in seven years. Recent Joint UN Action Plan on HIV/AIDS (UNAIDS, 2006) statistics estimate that approximately 5.5 million South Africans are infected with HIV, 14.8% of whom are young people between the ages of 15–24 years. These statistics indicate one of the largest numbers of individuals living with the virus in a single country.

The increase in HIV infections among the youth has occurred in spite of their knowledge of the disease and the many campaigns that have been mounted to halt the spread of the disease. Some of these campaigns have been mounted by the government. Government strategies have entailed, among other things, restructuring of the way in which HIV/AIDS is taught in schools, and intervention programmes and campaigns through the mass media. Some of the intervention programmes implemented by the government are loveLife (a national HIV/AIDS prevention programme for youth) and Khomanani (an HIV/AIDS and TB campaign). Globally, programmes that emphasise the need for greater awareness of HIV/AIDS and preventive measures have also been introduced. One programme introduced globally, and also in South Africa, was the three-pronged strategy for prevention of HIV infection known as the ABC approach, with the 'A' referring to abstinence, the 'B' to being faithful to a single (and uninfected) partner and the 'C' to condom use (Bankole, 2004). Despite this, youth remain the fastest-growing prevalence group in the country, hence the need to find out their understanding of and attitudes towards risk and sexual practice in the context of HIV/AIDS.

A study by Bradshaw (2004) show that young people in South Africa reported HIV/AIDS to be the biggest problem facing them and their communities, and many of them knew someone who had died of AIDS. But despite this, most of the respondents in Bradshaw et al's study did not consider themselves as being at risk of contracting the disease, including those who were already infected.

Methodology

As already pointed out, this study aimed at gaining an understanding of youth's conceptions of risk in the context of HIV/AIDS. Since the study sought to understand rather than prove the existence of the phenomenon under scrutiny, a qualitative methodological approach seemed more appropriate and useful. According to Goodwin and Goodwin (1996), qualitative research is particularly useful for ascertaining respondents' thoughts, perceptions, feelings and retrospective accounts of events, giving the reader a clear understanding of their conceptions of the world around them.

Within this qualitative framework, a phenomenological approach was most appropriate: 'Phenomenology is a method of philosophical inquiry, involving the systematic investigation of consciousness' (Seale, 2004). It allows for the study of people's understandings of a phenomenon and the detailed descriptions of their experiences and how subjects make sense of them (Babbie, 1999). In the present study, a phenomenological approach allowed for a deep understanding of youths' knowledge of HIV/AIDS, and their attitudes and behaviours in this regard.

Sampling strategy

Four schools were used in the study. The sampling of these schools occurred in two phases. The first phase was purposive, in that all the schools in the Cape Metropole area were grouped into the four different racial categories[1] that defined the way in which education was provided prior to the demise of apartheid in 1994. This phase was used to group schools into different racial and socioeconomic categories. In the second phase, simple random sampling was used to select the schools. One school from each of the four racial categories was randomly selected. The selection took into account aspects like race, religion, geographic origin of learners and their membership of local communities, socioeconomic status of school and communities, mobility of teachers and learners, ethnicity, and language.

Once the research process had begun, it became clear that one of the selected schools was facing many difficulties and the safety of the researcher was a concern. Gaining access to both the school and the respondents became difficult. For example, there was a suicide, gang-related violence and police involvement at the school on just one of the days that one of the authors visited the school. As a result of these factors, this school was dropped from the study and another school was selected.

[1] 'white', 'Indian', 'coloured' and 'black' schools.

Table 8.1 below gives a brief overview of the schools selected. Included too is the grade selected and the data collection methods used with each sample of learners. The four secondary schools are Bridgeview, Greenbelt, Meadowrise and Summerville High Schools.[2]

Table 8.1: Overview of schools, method of data collection and number of participants

Name of school	Bridgeview High School	Greenbelt High School	Meadowrise High School	Summerville High School
Grade	10	10	10	10
Questionnaire	One grade 10 class (35 participants)	One grade 10 class (36 participants)	One grade 10 class (45 participants)	One grade 10 class (25 participants)
Focus group discussions	10 learners	10 learners	10 learners	10 learners
Individual interviews	9 of the 10 learners from the focus group discussion (one learner declined to take part in the interview)	All 10 learners from the focus group discussion	All 10 learners from the focus group discussion	No interviews conducted[4]

Bridgeview High School is a former model C school.[3] It is a dual-medium school with learners able to take classes in either English or Afrikaans, depending on their mother tongue. The school draws pupils from a range of socioeconomic backgrounds; however, the majority of learners were middle-class. The class sizes were on average 35 pupils per class, and each pupil had a desk, chair and his/her own textbooks. All the pupils interviewed lived with one or both of their parents and family members, mostly in a house or duplex with a garden.

Greenbelt High School is an English-medium coeducational secondary school in a predominantly Muslim community. The majority of the pupils and teachers were coloured, and although it was an English-medium school, many of the learners spoke Afrikaans as their mother tongue. There were approximately 30 learners per class, each of whom had a desk and a chair, but often they had to share textbooks. In general, it drew children from both low- and middle-class socioeconomic backgrounds. The majority of the learners lived in the surrounding suburbs in homes or flats with their parents, family or extended family members.

Meadowrise High School was a coeducational secondary school in a township. It was previously under the Department of Education and Training (which catered for the education of black people) and had predominantly Xhosa- and Afrikaans-speaking learners.

2 These are pseudonyms. For confidentiality reasons, the schools' true names could not be used.

3 Model C schools were schools that were set aside for the exclusive use of white students, which, upon the introduction of the 'open' schools policy in 1990, were allowed to convert themselves to semi-private and semi-state schools and enrol black learners.

On average there were 40–50 learners per class who often had to share desks, chairs and textbooks. The relationship between teachers and learners was very formal and some of the teachers had strict classroom management techniques where pupils were forbidden to talk unless spoken to. This is, however, a generalisation and not all classes were as strictly managed. The majority of the learners came from a low socioeconomic background, and many were the first in their families to go to secondary school. Many of them lived in one-roomed informal dwellings, with no running water a shared outside toilet and no electricity. In some cases there were up to 11 family members or extended family members living together in a one-roomed house. Most of the learners walked to school, many over long distances, and a few came to school by mini-bus taxi.

Summerville High School was an all-girls, Anglican, English-medium independent school. It drew its children from a predominantly middle- to upper-class background. The school offers scholarships and bursaries to previously disadvantaged students; therefore, there were also learners from very poor backgrounds in the school. It also had a boarding house and drew learners from over 20 different countries. It was, therefore, culturally very rich and diverse. The maximum class size permitted was 25 learners per class. Each learner had a desk, chair and her own textbooks, as well as many other teaching aids. The majority of the learners were from wealthy backgrounds living in large, modern homes, and they would be dropped off at school in cars by their parents.

The descriptions of the four schools above provide a preview of the contexts within which the learners operated and made meaning of their lives. It is important to take cognisance of these different contexts in understanding the significance of this study.

As Table 8.1 shows, only one grade 10 class in each of the four schools was involved in the study. Grade 10 teachers assisted in selecting the class that was involved in the study. The choice of grade 10 learners was informed by the fact that most of them were in the adolescent age category, as the average age of grade 10 learners in South African schools is approximately 15–16 years. This age was considered appropriate for investigating perceptions of risk in the context of HIV/AIDS, as the learners were adolescents and likely to be either considering or in sexual relationships. The table also shows the three methods of data collection that were utilised, ie questionnaire, focus group discussions (FGD) and individual interviews.

Theoretical framework

The study was underpinned by theories that sought to explain the construction of youth identities and the understandings of risk among young people, especially adolescents. Constructions of identity are complex and can be understood from many different theoretical perspectives. Psychologists and, more specifically, developmental and psychoanalytical psychologists such as Freud, Piaget and Erikson see identity construction as stage specific and intrinsic to the individual. For example, Erikson's (1968) psychoanalytical theory argues that although development and therefore identity construction

[4] Individual interviews were not conducted at Summerville because it was nearing examination time at the time of the study and the school declined to allow the learners to participate in the individual interviews. The school thought that the interviews would distract the learners from preparing for the examinations.

happen in stages, a key characteristic of the self is that selfhood is personally created, interpretively elaborated and interpersonally constructed. In other words, the individual is part of the process of constructing his/her own identity.

Freud describes adolescence as the puberty or genital stage brought about by the biological maturation of the individual's reproductive system (Muus, 1988). He characterises this stage by a rapid increase in sexual tensions demanding gratification. These sexual needs and fantasies become more explicitly concerned with tension release and later the sexual union of male and female. Freud further claims that these inclinations are restrained by social demands and the individual's adaptation to the moral values of society and the norms of his/her community (Muus, 1988). This creates conflict within the individual, as often sexual desires are not met due to societal demands and views of appropriateness. Often gratification is sought, resulting in feelings of guilt by the individual, due to him/her being caught between moral pressures and the need to fulfil desires. This produces conflict, turmoil and disequilibrium (Muus, 1988). These conflicts can be internal or external, eg within the individual or between parents and their children. Freud's ideas help one to understand youth identity, as they see youth as being a difficult phase in a person's life, due to the many changes not only in one's body at this time, but the difficulties in trying to establish a more adult identity as well.

Erikson (1968), a developmental theorist, focuses on eight stages of development, distinguishing identity formation during adolescence from similar phases during infancy and childhood. Erikson (1968) argues that identity has to be searched for and that its creation is a conscious process. It is not given to the individual by society, nor does it appear as a maturation phenomenon such as that described by Freud. Rather, Erikson argues that identity must be acquired through sustained individual effort. When discussing youth's search for personal identity, he describes it as the process of forming a personal ideology or philosophy of life that gives the individual a frame of reference for evaluating events. Erikson emphasises the role that peers have in shaping adolescent identity. He describes how childhood dependency on parents later becomes the adolescent's dependency on his or her peers (Erikson, 1968).

Giddens' (1987) theory of structuration provides an analytical framework for understanding youth in a modern context. This theory focuses on how we draw on external things when constructing our identities and internal things to make choices. Giddens unpacks the relationships between individuals and the conditions around them. He postulates that the connection between structure and agency is a fundamental element of social theory, and that these two factors cannot be conceived of apart from one another. At a basic level, this means that people make society, but at the same time are constrained by it; ie structures are created, maintained and changed through actions, while actions are given meaningful form only through the background of the structure. Individuals have scope as to the choices they make within these structures, and it is the structures that provide the range of choices for us. The two work together simultaneously (Giddens, 1991).

Giddens' theory of structuration highlights the importance of not only how the individual perceives him- or herself in the modern world, but of how the context in which one lives contributes to shaping our social realms and thus has an effect on the nature of our choice making. Giddens' theory helps to equip one to talk about risk and more specifically youth and risk in a modern context. Psychological theorists such as Freud, Piaget and Erikson do not talk about risk specifically, and one can only base assumptions about their understandings regarding youth and risk on their references to the phase of adolescence described in their theories. For example, Freud's focus on youth's biological and sexual desires gives rise to a possible argument that youth put themselves at risk, particularly sexually related risk (HIV and sexually transmitted diseases — STDs), as their urges to fulfil biological desires may override logical rational thought and the need to protect themselves. It would assume that choices are made irrationally, based on desire rather than the fear of risks and consequences. A feeling of guilt or rational thought may come later, but initial decisions are not necessarily made logically.

It is evident that understanding how youth construct their identities is very complex. Also, youth identities are not fixed, as suggested by developmental and psychoanalytical theories. Giddens' theory is the most useful for this study as it recognises the complex nature of identity construction and the many influences that affect this process. Giddens' theory is therefore important in understanding the relationship between youth and how they go about making decisions in the context of a modern high-risk HIV/AIDS environment. For example, when understanding youth in such a context in South Africa, one cannot ignore, among other things, the cultural and religious beliefs affecting youth, the range of communities and socioeconomic levels from which they come, and how each particular context will have a profound influence not only in how each individual constructs his/her own identity, but in the nature of their beliefs and understandings and therefore their choice making.

What follows is a discussion of the understanding of risk by the learners in the four schools (Bridgeview, Greenbelt, Meadowrise and Summerville) in the context of HIV/AIDS. The first part of the discussion focuses on the learners' definitions of risk, followed by an examination of notions of invincibility and invulnerability to HIV infection held by the learners. The final part of the discussion focuses on condom use.

Main findings

Learners' conceptions of risk

Conceptions of risk were, as the following suggests, embedded in the deeper meanings associated with risk and risky behaviour in the communities in which the learners made meaning for themselves. The definitional meaning of risk as they understood it influenced their perceptions of and responses to questions about HIV infection.

Learners' definitions of risk

The respondents defined risk according to their chances of falling pregnant, being in an accident, and getting HIV or other STDs. A female respondent from Bridgeview High School said, 'risk is how likely you are to fall pregnant'. A male informant from Greenbelt High School said, 'risk is the chances people have of something bad happening to them, like a car accident or a drug overdose', while a respondent from Summerville High School said, 'risk can refer to many things like someone's likelihood of getting HIV, falling pregnant or being in an accident'.

In most cases, the respondents saw these categories of risk (falling pregnant, contracting HIV, etc) as being outside of themselves and problematic only for others.

Most of the respondents referred to risk in the third person, using words such as 'other', 'them', 'people' and 'someone'. It can therefore be said that the majority of the respondents held views of invincibility and that they thought they themselves were not at risk of any of the things they mentioned.

However, the respondents from Meadowrise High School, many of whom had had a family member or friend affected or infected by HIV/AIDS, thought that their chances of getting the disease were slightly higher than people living in more urban, wealthy areas, where the living conditions were better. Seven out of the ten learners from Summerville High School thought they were least likely to be at risk and that people living in poorer areas, with less education and poor access to good medical care, would be at higher risk. However, some of the learners in the same school disagreed. One respondent argued:

> AIDS, car accidents, sexually transmitted diseases and such things, do not discriminate like people do. We are all equally at risk and it is often the choices we make that put us at risk rather than where we live.

The respondents also defined risk according to degrees of risk; in other words, what they feared most and felt they were most at risk of. In all four schools, there was a greater fear of becoming pregnant (for girls) or impregnating a girl (in the case of the male respondents), than there was of contracting HIV or other STDs. One respondent put it this way: 'I am far more afraid of falling pregnant than getting HIV. HIV is uncommon in my community, whereas pregnancy can easily happen'. Not only did the informants see pregnancy as a greater risk, but they saw the possibility of pregnancy as being far more likely than contracting an STD or HIV.

Another factor that featured when talking about risk was that of knowing one's HIV status. All except five of the informants said they would be anxious about having an HIV test, even if they knew they had nothing to worry about. Here the use of the word 'knew' is interesting, as it implies that they know they have nothing to worry about. One respondent stated: 'I'd rather be "status free" than know I may have HIV. If I don't know my status I can say I am negative!' This attitude says a lot about these youths' conceptions and perceptions of risk, as denying one's status is to deny one is at risk and that one could be putting others at risk too.

Four points may be drawn from the respondents' definition and understanding of risk, especially with regard to HIV/AIDS. The first is that those who have 'experienced' the disease through friends and family who are affected and infected by the virus acknowledge that they could be at risk of being infected. They understand that HIV/AIDS is not a disease for 'other' people, but people like themselves. The second point is the identification and association of HIV/AIDS with certain kinds of people, eg poor people. The notion expressed by some respondents that only poor people were at risk of contracting HIV also introduces a class dimension into the construction of the risk of contracting the disease. Such notions encourage the thinking that people outside the 'at risk class' are not in danger of being infected.

The third is the inherent contradiction in some notions of risk of infection. The section of the respondents that considered pregnancy as their major risk captures this contradiction. They seemed to be oblivious of the fact that both pregnancy and HIV/AIDS infection are usually consequences of unprotected sex. The last point refers to complacency regarding the respondents' HIV status, with many of them taking for granted that they were HIV-negative. These four points suggest that the majority of the respondents generally considered HIV/AIDS as being a problem of other people.

Invincibility/invulnerability to HIV infection

As alluded to above, there seemed to be some general patterns as to how the respondents conceived the risk of contracting HIV/AIDS, irrespective of their gender, race or geographic location. The majority of respondents held views of invincibility, thinking that they were not at risk and that they were invulnerable to HIV infection. There were, however, nodes of difference, and these related directly to individual differences and contexts such as class, religious inclination, family background, geographic location and personality.

In both the focus group discussions and the individual interviews, there was a sense of invincibility among most of the learners in all four schools. There was a resounding attitude that, to quote one learner: 'It [HIV/AIDS] will never happen to me.' There was no sense of fear of HIV/AIDS infection, even in those communities where the learners had family members who were infected with the disease or had even lost family members to it. Surprisingly, there was still a sense that it would never happen to them. One learner at Summerville High School said: 'Even when I am drunk I know what I am doing and I always feel in control.'

Another opinion that was expressed by most of the learners with little or no experience of or exposure (through an infected friend or family member) to the disease was that until they had experience of the disease, they would not fear it or be wary of it. A learner from Summerville High School said: 'Nobody I know personally or hang around with has the disease, therefore how could I get it?' This once again shows this learner's sense of invincibility and lack of fear of being at risk. In her opinion, HIV is still a disease 'out there' and not within her community. A respondent from Bridgeview High School said:

> They must stop showing us poor, starving, sick black people. Show us our 'own' people dying and then we'll maybe change our attitudes and behaviour. What have we got to be scared of, when the only people we hear about with the disease are of a different race and from a different area?

Perhaps discouraged by the predominant notions of invulnerability to HIV infection, one girl from Summerville High School commented:

> I think people will only be scared of AIDS in about 20 years time, when they actually see what it is doing to our people and more so the effects it is having on our country and its economy. We need to see the effects of HIV/AIDS, like we do with pregnancy when one of our friends falls pregnant.

Some respondents, especially at Summerville High School, rejected the notion that HIV/AIDS did not exist in their communities. A respondent from the school stated: 'I know AIDS must exist in my community, but people hide it and carry on as normal, so it is difficult to believe.' Another said: 'I'm sure AIDS must exist in this community, but I have never been directly exposed to it.' The dominant notion that HIV/AIDS is not a problem in the Summerville community suggests a lack of readiness by this community to confront the disease. This lack of readiness seems to be informed by notions of invulnerability and the perceptions of the disease as belonging elsewhere — as a problem of other people who are not like 'us'. The lack of acceptance of the disease as a problem in this community could also be linked with stigma. Since the dominant notion is that it is a disease of other people, 'hiding it' could be seen as an attempt to avoid being seen as the 'others' whom the disease infects.

Generally, the attitude of most of the learners in all four schools was that of invincibility, and they did not consider themselves to be at any particular risk of contracting HIV. All except three of the informants had little fear of the disease — even those with direct exposure to it through a friend or family member. And even in cases where the respondents *did* have experience of the disease, fulfilling their own sexual desires, 'becoming a man' by being sexually active and the fear of pregnancy tended to outweigh their fears about the risks of HIV/AIDS. According to most of the respondents, the people who are at risk of contracting HIV are, among others, babies of HIV-positive breastfeeding mothers, people living with HIV-positive people, poor people with little education, people who get raped and children who are sexually abused. From this data, for the most part, youth perceived vulnerability to HIV infection as belonging to others rather than themselves. There was a sense that they were in control of their own lives and that nothing could happen to them.

The perception of invulnerability to HIV infection by the learners is consistent with the findings of other studies on the subject, such as Bradshaw et al's (2004). This study shows that although young people reported HIV/AIDS to be the biggest problem facing them and their communities and 45% of the respondents reported that they personally knew someone who had died of AIDS, the majority of them did not consider themselves personally at risk of contracting HIV. It is reasonable to conclude that if the youth do not feel at risk of contracting HIV, then they will not see the need to protect themselves against it.

Although reducing the number of sexual partners is key to minimising the risk of HIV infection (Bradshaw et al, 2004), only six of the respondents considered this to be a viable option. For many of them, serial monogamy was not of particular concern, and their attitude was that being young was a chance to experiment by having many sexual relationships and having fun. The six respondents who considered serial monogamy as important in reducing the risk of HIV infection had strong religious beliefs; ie standpoint on monogamy was not necessarily motivated by their perceptions of risk of HIV infection, but rather their value systems.

From the discussion, it is clear that notions of youth invincibility and invulnerability to HIV infection are complex. There is no particular way of understanding why even though the youth engaged in risky behaviour (eg having multiple sexual partners), the majority of them did not consider themselves as being at risk of infection. Also, from a common-sense perspective, one would imagine that those who had encountered the disease through infected friends and family would not hold perceptions of invulnerability. But, as the discussion has shown, this was not always the case. To add to the complexity, there were those who attributed their perceptions of invincibility to the fact that none of those close to them (a friend or relative) had ever been infected with HIV/

AIDS. Overall, it can be concluded that a general account of youth invincibility is not possible. It varies among individuals, communities and contexts.

Condom use

The learners' attitudes towards condom use also varied enormously, but were fairly community specific. In cases where informants felt that condom use was important, the main reason for their use was as protection against pregnancy rather than against HIV or other STDs. None of the learners indicated that condom use was firstly for the prevention of HIV/AIDS. This was always an afterthought. An informant from Bridgeview High School said: 'Girls and boys are scared of pregnancy and [irrespective of] what other people may think, HIV/AIDS often does not even enter their thoughts'. A respondent from Greenbelt High School added:

> [Young] people are far more concerned about falling pregnant than getting AIDS. The problem is that they know they can always go to the chemist and get the 'morning after pill' to prevent pregnancy, and therefore the necessity for condom use often falls away.

Considering that the learners did not always use condoms to prevent pregnancy (some used contraceptive pills, among other methods), it may be concluded that their risk of infection with HIV/AIDS and other STDs was quite high.

Some of the respondents, particularly at Meadowrise High School, also had negative attitudes towards condom use due to certain beliefs. All the boys, as well as most of the girls at this school had the belief, as one of the learners put it, that: 'Sex is not sex if you use a condom.' Another respondent stated: 'If a boy uses a condom, it makes you less of a "man" and that is seen as being very important'. Also, almost all the respondents at Meadowrise High School held the view that sex needed to be 'skin on skin' to be enjoyable.

Another belief that prevented some of the learners from using condoms and promoted their sense of invincibility was the belief that one could not get AIDS from a virgin, therefore condom use with a virgin was not important. Two male respondents from Meadowrise High School also believed that if you do not have sexual intercourse for seven months, you once again become a virgin, and in this case, condom use is once again unnecessary. Seemingly, these respondents were prepared to enter into high-risk sexual behaviour rather than protecting themselves. These beliefs appeared to be deeply embedded cultural understandings about the use of condoms and, therefore, overrode any fear of risk and fed into the culture of invincibility. For these respondents, condom use was not a viable option for the above-mentioned reasons, suggesting that a sense of invincibility or invulnerability to infection by HIV overrode the risk and fear of contracting the disease or other STDs.

Other reasons advanced by respondents for not using condoms were that condoms were expensive and it was embarrassing to purchase them. A respondent from Bridgeview High School said: 'Using condoms makes sex an expensive habit'. Condoms were also frowned upon because they allegedly had a bad odour, inhibited pleasure and were inconvenient. There was also the notion that condom use would imply a lack of trust in a (sexual) partner. It may be argued that these perceptions about condoms inhibited their use. Denzin and Lincoln (1998) point out that 'in order for condoms to be effective against HIV infection, they must be used consistently and correctly'. Young people seem to be aware of this, yet their behaviour patterns do not reflect this. Bradshaw et al (2004), and Skinner and Mfecane (2004) make the point that many young people still held the misconception that using a condom meant that one did not trust one's sexual partner and that there was almost a universal perception that condoms were not acceptable at both a cultural and personal level. Skinner and Mfecane (2004) further state that the youth know about HIV/AIDS, how it is transmitted and how to protect themselves, but there are too many pressures in terms of prevailing sexual norms for condoms to be widely used. This was also confirmed in this study.

Overall, the majority of the learners felt that their chances of contracting HIV or an STD were so small that they would rather not use condoms. All of the above evidence shows that the learners' sense of invincibility was greater than their conceptions of risk and fear of the disease.

Discussion

As has been shown in the preceding sections, the majority of respondents did not consider themselves personally at risk of contracting HIV/AIDS. This is consistent with other studies such as Bradshaw et al's (2004). The general feeling among many of the respondents was that HIV/AIDS was still a disease 'out there', a disease of other people, and that until they begin to see its effects on their communities, close friends and family members, it would not be something they truly feared. Given, as was shown in the discussion, that some communities (eg Summerville) did not acknowledge the existence of the disease among them, it is not suprising that the youth in such communities would hold perceptions of invincibility and invulnerability to HIV/AIDS infection for a long time. A more worrying phenomenon was in cases where the respondents had experienced the disease through an infected and affected friend or family member, yet they still held perceptions of invincibility with regard to infection.

The general impression from the study's findings is that being popular among their peers, fulfilling their own sexual desires, 'becoming a man' by being sexually active and the fear of pregnancy tended to outweigh the respondents' fears about the risks of HIV/AIDS. Perceptions of invincibility and invulnerability to HIV infection among young people are a formidable challenge to positive behaviour change and efforts to prevent HIV/AIDS infections among the youth. Therefore, concerted efforts need to be made to dispel these perceptions.

Another important finding was the negative attitudes towards condom use. Many of the respondents felt that if one used a contraceptive pill or injection, there was little need for condom use, as the chances of falling pregnant were very small. For these informants, HIV/AIDS was not considered as a necessary concern, as they did not consider themselves to be at risk and therefore had no reason to use condoms. Thus, the majority of the respondents were more concerned about the risk of becoming pregnant than of contracting HIV/AIDS.

Condom use was unpopular with the respondents for several reasons, ie that it inhibited pleasure and that condoms were expensive, inconvenient, odorous and embarrassing to purchase. Many respondents also held the view that suggesting condom use to a partner implied a lack of trust in the partner. These reasons inhibited condom use and also suggest that where they were used, it was only irregularly. The negative attitudes towards condom use by the respondents support the observation by Skinner and Mfecane (2004) that there was an almost universal perception that condoms were not acceptable at both the cultural and personal levels.

As was argued in the theoretical framework, the construction of youth identities and how youth make choices are complex processes. Giddens' theory postulates that the choices people, as agents, make are the result of a multiplicity of factors. From the findings of this study, it is clear that these factors bring about unpredictable responses. Thus, the relationship among the various factors and the responses by agents is non-linear and unpredictable. A good example is the perception of invincibility and invulnerability to HIV/AIDS infection by some respondents because of the belief that their community was not at risk. The flip side of this perception is that respondents who had experienced the disease in their communities would consider themselves as being vulnerable to infection. But the findings of this study show the opposite, as respondents who had friends and family members who were affected and infected by HIV/AIDS also held perceptions of invulnerability to infection. It appears that the magnitude of the influence of other factors, such as the macho phenomenon, that encouraged the feeling of invulnerability to HIV/AIDS infection was greater than the expected result of having an infected and affected friend or family member, ie considering oneself as vulnerable.

It cannot, therefore, be taken for granted that certain factors have greater influence on youth's perceptions of risk of HIV/AIDS infection than others. It is imperative that key factors, as viewed by the youth themselves, be identified and addressed appropriately. Some of the factors, for instance, those that prevent youth from using condoms, seem mundane, and one could easily dismiss them as irrelevant. This would be a mistake, as these have been identified by the agents as influencing their agency in very particular ways.

Overall, Giddens' (1987; 1991) theory looks at the modern subject living in a modern world and how he/she has to make choices, knowing that all choices have consequences and involve risk. He concludes that we live in highly conflictual spaces and have to make choices involving risk. It is therefore inevitable that, at times, poor choices will be made. This was evident from the findings in that many of the choices youth make about behaviour involved risk and in many cases poor choices were made, such as the choice to have unprotected sex.

It is clear from the study's findings that the risk Giddens refers to is not necessarily acknowledged by all agents. The youth, as illustrated in this study, tend to have a sense of invincibility, ignoring the risk factors involved in their decision-making processes. This shows the difficulty many youth experience in seeing the relationship between their actions and the possible consequences of those actions.

Conclusion

As the foregoing discussion has shown, although HIV/AIDS remains one of the biggest challenges facing adolescents in South Africa, the perception of risk of infection by many of them contradicts messages about prevention and the spread of the disease.

Many of the adolescents in this study have illusions of invulnerability to HIV infection. They are not afraid of getting HIV, and, to a large degree, have the attitude: 'It can't happen to me'. It is interesting that the fear of falling pregnant superseded that of contracting HIV.

The reasons for the prevailing sense of invulnerability to HIV infection by the respondents in the study are varied. For some, it was because they had not 'experienced' the disease through an infected close friend or relative; and for some non-black students, it is partly because the disease is usually presented (especially in the media) as a problem facing black people. Interestingly, even adolescents who had 'experienced' the disease through infected close relatives and friends still held notions of invincibility. Unfortunately, the adolescents' illusions of invulnerability seemed to influence risky sexual behaviours such as having multiple sexual partners and non-use of condoms.

Overall, the relationships between individuals (adolescents) and the conditions (context) around them, as postulated by Giddens (1987), are important in understanding both the constructions of risk of HIV infection and formulating effective preventive strategies. In this study, the context of the adolescents is shaped by, among other things, their socioeconomic backgrounds, race and cultural dispositions.

Chapter 9

Marit Petersen
Oslo University College

Cultural Practices, Gender and HIV/AIDS: A Study of Young Women's Sexual Positioning in the Context of HIV/AIDS in South Africa

Introduction

This chapter examines the ways in which young women and men interpret and enact gender roles in general, and more specifically within sexual relationships. It explores how gender dynamics influence sexual behaviour in relation to the risk of HIV infection among adolescents in two different communities in the Cape Town area. Further, it examines the social and cultural practices and attitudes that shape youth's sexual identity construction in relation to HIV/AIDS. The intersection between cultural context or cultural beliefs and the effectiveness of HIV/AIDS intervention programmes in Cape Town schools is also explored.

HIV/AIDS in South Africa

South Africa has experienced one of the most rapid growths in HIV infections in the world. Towards the end of 2003 estimates showed that 5.3 million South Africans were HIV positive (UNAIDS, 2006; Karim, 2005). This disease is thus one of the major threats to social, economic and political well-being in the country. The reasons for the rapid spread of HIV in South Africa are many and complex. They include high levels of poverty and income inequality, high levels of other sexually transmitted infections (STIs), a predominant patriarchal system that ascribes a low status to women, sexual activity at early ages, multiple sexual partners, unprotected sex, sexual violence, and lack of communication about sexuality between parents and children. South Africa's HIV conundrum is also linked with the migrant labour system and the disruption of family and community life (Walker, Reid & Cornell, 2004; Karim, 2005). Many interventions have been implemented to try and arrest the disease. In spite of these interventions, ranging from educational programmes to extensive media campaigns, there has been very little effect on the spread of the disease (Baxen & Breidlid, 2004).

Missing from the literature is a more nuanced understanding of how gender roles are negotiated in intimate contexts and how such negotiation influences sexual risk interactions between women and men. Underemphasised in the literature is how social, economic and cultural factors in particular settings shape sex and sexuality. Parker (in Kelly & Ntlabati, 2002:47) explains:

> Sexual desire has been treated, in many ways, as a kind of given, and the social and cultural factors shaping sexual experience in different settings have largely been ignored, even when lip service has been paid to their potential importance .... Emphasis, instead, has been placed largely on individual determinants of sexual behaviour and behaviour change, and the diverse, cultural, economic, and political factors potentially influencing or even shaping sexual experience have more often than not been ignored.

Cultural and contextual conditions should be appreciated far more, because they play an important and often decisive role in how people make meaning of their lives in general, and in particular, how negotiations and decisions relating to sex are made. Nattrass (2004) emphasises that sexual cultures in South Africa are an important dimension in the country's HIV pandemic. According to her, gender inequality; sexual violence; fatalistic attitudes; and, in some communities, pressure to prove fertility contribute to a high-risk environment. Cultural practices and attitudes towards sex play a significant role in increasing the vulnerability of women to infection. In many societies, women lack control over their bodies and, for the most part, over decisions about their lives. They are usually socialised from an early age to be subordinate and submissive to men (Ouzgane & Morrell, 2005). Socially and culturally promoted male dominance, where women's rights over their own bodies are compromised, often makes negotiations in relationships difficult. A substantial body of South African research describes the importance of gender dynamics, including violence against women within sexual relationships as factors underlying HIV risk (Wood & Jewkes 1997b; 1998; 2001; LeClerc-Madlala, 2002a; O'Sullivan et al, 2006; Karim, 2005). Women are often unable to insist on condom use in relationships where they are not only aware of, but have evidence of, infidelity. This represents a dilemma resulting in sexual risk in that women often find it difficult, if not impossible, to negotiate safer sex practices in abusive relationships.

Mathews (2005:151) points out that it is important for prevention initiatives in South Africa to

> follow theoretical approaches that do take account of the broader social and environmental factors — where the premise is that the collective health of communities can be enhanced by processes, structures and policies that foster individual health-promoting actions or reduce or eliminate health hazards in the social and physical environment.

This chapter reports on a study that examined the contextual factors that shape sexual behaviour particularly among girls, and the preventive steps taken by the authorities. Although a number of studies (eg Baxen & Breidlid, 2004) describe South African cultural beliefs that have a bearing on sexual behaviour, the impact of social and cultural beliefs on sexual behaviour and negotiation is often a matter of conjecture. An examination of the deeply held beliefs and practices about sexuality, as well as the everyday sexual practices among youth in some schools in South Africa, is, therefore, the main focus of this chapter.

Choice of site and schools

Two schools that participated in the larger research project described in the introduction to this book served as primary sites for data reported in this chapter.

The first, Masani Secondary School, is situated in a predominantly black, poor, working-class township and the other, Birkenhead Secondary School, in a middle-class, predominantly white suburb.[1] The demographics of these two schools are worth noting. Masani caters for predominantly Xhosa-speaking, black[2] students, while Birkenhead, a historically Afrikaans-speaking monolingual school, now has a combination of Afrikaans and English speakers. While most of the student population is white and middle-class, the school does attract children from coloured working- and middle-class backgrounds. These, however, are in the minority.

The rationale for the choice of schools was the variation in HIV prevalence (Gouws & Karim, 2005; Breidlid, 2005) among the two communities. A district survey in the Western Cape in 2004 revealed that the black townships of Gugulethu, where Masani is located, had an HIV prevalence rate of 28.1%, far above other districts in the Western Cape (Breidlid, 2005). Furthermore, HIV/AIDS has proven to vary in relation to socioeconomic status and education (Breidlid, 2005). It made sense, therefore, to include a middle-class community where the prevalence rate is lower than the provincial rate of 12%.

Masani Secondary

The school lies in a community that experiences high rates of unemployment. Thus, learners at Masani live in poor conditions. The school is in desperate need of repair. Classes are overcrowded (40–50 learners per class) and the school has no grounds for extra-mural activities. The school has a policy of allowing learners to leave the school grounds during breaks to go home for meals. It is not uncommon, therefore, to experience a drop in attendance after both school breaks. Because the researcher was only able to communicate in English, children who participated at both schools were required to be proficient in English.

Birkenhead Secondary

This is a well-established and materially well-resourced school. It has sprawling sports grounds, with sports participation a compulsory feature of the school curriculum. The school has mini-vans to transport learners to various sporting events. It has an average of 25–35 children in a class and has a sizeable population (about 20 of 70) of teachers who hold governing body positions.[3] This enables the school to maintain smaller classes. The many displays in the foyer, administrative section and principal's office illustrate that academic achievement and sports are privileged in this school. Learners are respectful and greet visitors as a courtesy. Unlike at Masani, this school was orderly and no children were seen outside of classes during teaching time.

The background of the communities and schools is important, as it locates the study in different socioeconomic contexts that influence understandings of and responses to gender and HIV.

---

1 The two schools are each given a pseudonym in order to protect their identities.

2 Though problematic and controversial, these terms are still in use in South Africa. African or black person, coloured person and white person were the terminologies used by my respondents; hence I chose to use them in the study.

3 This means that teachers' salaries are paid by the school through school fees and other fund-raising activities.

Methodological considerations

The aim of the study was to generate a holistic and in-depth understanding of how the respondents' sociocultural contexts gave meaning to and shaped their sexual choices and thus their HIV vulnerability. The data collection was in two parts. While the main study was qualitative and interpretive, a questionnaire was administered to one class of grade 11 learners at each of the schools. This was to ascertain their knowledge of HIV/AIDS. For the main study, data collection was primarily through individual semi-structured interviews, researcher field notes and informants' diaries.

Ten female respondents aged between 16 and 18 were selected from each school. To triangulate the data and verify the perspectives and experiences of the female respondents, five males of the same age, as well as five parents from each school, were selected to participate in the study. The sample thus comprised 40 participants.

In-depth semi-structured interviews formed the basis of the study. According to Kvale (2001:21), the purpose of in-depth interviews is 'to collect descriptions of the interviewee's life world with a view to interpreting the described phenomena'. The main advantage of this research strategy is that it offers more comprehensive answers from the participants and it allows for greater flexibility. An interview guide was used during the interviews. A tape recorder was used to record the interviews after permission was sought from the interviewees to do so.

The questionnaire contained questions about the knowledge base of youth, while the interviews of parents and male respondents focused on views on sexuality and the role of females in relationships.

Theoretical framework

Two main theories were employed in the study: script theory (Simon & Gagnon 1987; Gagnon & Parker, 1995; Laumann & Gagnon, 1995; Gagnon & Simon, 2005) and sex role theory (Connell, 1987). Different socialisation theories and South African research on youth and sexuality were also utilised in the analysis.

Script theory

Script theory provides a useful framework to analyse and understand the social construction of gender roles. The great variation in sexual expression indicates that sexuality is learned and internalised through social processes. From an early stage, human beings learn the 'acceptable' norms for where, when and with whom they can live out their physical sexuality. This indicates that sexual behaviour may vary within and between countries, communities and cultures and during different historical periods (Connell, 1987; Kelly & Ntlabati, 2002).

Gagnon and Parker (1995) use the term 'gender' to refer to the social construction of roles, responsibilities and obligations associated with being a man or woman. Gender roles are culturally defined sets of behaviours that differentiate maleness and femaleness and are incorporated into 'scripts', which are culturally stereotyped, sequential interactions between two people who are responding to each other's cues and actions (Gagnon & Simon, 2005). Scripts characterise the ways in which gender, sexuality and relationships are negotiated at the three interrelated levels of mutually shared conventions: the cultural, interpersonal and individual levels (Laumann & Gagnon, 1995). The scenarios are descriptive: they specify 'acceptable' sexual behaviour, 'acceptable' partners and in which conditions sexuality can be expressed. Individual choices are thus a result of the individual's wishes put into a context with the cultural scenarios into which that individual has been socialised (Simon & Gagnon, 1987).

Script theory allows both inclusion of the social construction of gender roles and sexuality as well as analysis using the specific cultures and contexts that this study deals with. Moreover, the focus on male identity construction and 'hegemonic masculinity' (Connell, 1996; Cornwall & Lindisfarne, 1994; Mac an Ghaill, 1996) is of relevance in order to shed light on and complement the analysis of the female role — and indirectly the dynamics of the gender roles.

Sex role theory

Sex role theory is based on the idea of role learning, socialising and internalising. The main idea in the sex role paradigm is that men and women play roles decided in part by their sex (Connell, 1987). Such an approach to gender underlines that society's role expectations have an influence on how males and females reproduce their sexual identities. It also shapes their attitudes and subsequent behaviours. The individual's social position shows the importance of studying the interaction between people and the institutions responsible for teaching, the so-called agencies of socialisation (Connell, 1987). People at home and in school (including peers) have influence on the individual's cognitive and emotional development (Berndt, 1996; Bronfenbrenner, 1979). This dynamic is complex. Darnell and Höem (1996), though, underline the importance of the link between these two arenas as a decisive premise for the positive development of the individual, because knowledge is formed socially through a community of interests and values. According to Karim (2005), Campbell (2003) and Breidlid (2002), this feeling of community between home and school does not exist among the Xhosas in South Africa, but rather (as in other groups in South Africa) there is a tension between traditional cultural values and more modern perspectives in and through which young people are required to make a sexual identity particularly in relation to their risk of HIV/AIDS.

Main findings

Two themes frame the discussion in the main findings. The first focuses on the adequacy and sources of knowledge about sexuality and HIV/AIDS among the female respondents in the two schools in the study. The second describes how gender roles and sexual behaviour are shaped in the two communities and how this affects the experience of the female respondents.

Adequacy of knowledge about sexuality and HIV/AIDS

> It is important [to have] a pedagogy that is compatible with and includes the values and expectations of the students' cultural backgrounds. There has been provided evidence that culture does matter in classrooms and schools (Yamauchi & O'Donnell, 2005:6).

The Life Orientation learning area (which includes life-skills, HIV/AIDS and sex education) was introduced in 1998 as an important national prevention strategy in the South

African curriculum (known as C2005[4]). The aim is to adapt preventive sexual education for all ages and integrate it throughout the school system (DoE, 2003a).

Both the in-depth interviews and the questionnaire revealed that the factual knowledge of sexuality and HIV/AIDS prevention was high among the students from the two schools. Other studies in South Africa, though, have shown that there is great variation in knowledge and awareness of HIV/AIDS among adolescents. Such knowledge and awareness are partly hampered by a lack of reproductive health knowledge, as the information young people have is often unreliable and inaccurate (see, for instance, Harrison, 2005; Levine & Ross, 2002; Da Cruz, 2004).

Sources of knowledge about sexuality and HIV/AIDS

All the respondents in this study indicated that they received information about sexuality and HIV/AIDS mostly from their peers, the school and the media. A stark finding was the prevailing 'culture of silence' around sexuality and HIV/AIDS reported by students at Masani Secondary School. Almost all of them reported not discussing sex, HIV/AIDS or issues related to sexuality with their parents. This, according to them, was true even in the case of infection. A black female learner explained it in this way:

> I know and love someone with AIDS. It's a punishment and a prison so big. It's a disease that digs a grave for you whether you want to or not. People will treat you differently if you share your secret. They don't want to know you or have anything to do with you. They might say bad things about you behind your back. People are scared to be left alone. The parents of a friend of mine died because of AIDS. My friend didn't realise it until after they were dead.

The female respondents maintained that, in the learners' communities, it was often difficult to discuss or obtain information from people close to them, thus reinforcing a sense of shame at both the personal and institutional levels. This, as Kelly (2000) suggests, leads to stigma.

In contrast, the respondents at Birkenhead communicated more openly with their parents about sexuality, even though silence was also prevalent. According to DeLamater (1987), open dialogue in the homes often leads to less sexual risk taking among adolescents.

Even though knowledge is produced in many different arenas, it has been found that the knowledge produced in the homes and among peers has a major influence on adolescents' sexual behaviour. Davidson and Leslie (in Rodgers, 1996:89–90) point out that the influence of peer group and family lies mainly in the fact that 'the groups of which one is a member become a point of reference for the shaping of attitudes, values, and behaviour'.

Gender roles and sexual behaviour

The sex role theory connects social structure to the forming of personality (Connell, 1987) and explains why gender roles have different meanings in different societies and

[4] C2005 was revised in 2006. The result is a less cumbersome, more content-based national curriculum statement.

cultures at various times. This might explain the differences in the gender roles within the two contexts in the study. The gender roles at Masani seemed to be reproduced to reinforce hegemonic masculine and feminine identities, which, according to the sex role theory, is a situation where humans find themselves in stereotyped positions and play particular roles on the basis of their gender (Connell, 1987). In this environment, it was not uncommon for females to perceive their roles or positions as less important than those of men. They also perceived men as the decision makers. The following, by a black female in Masani, was a typical response:

> Mostly, the men make the decisions in a relationship. The girls most of the time let them do so, and often you can't do nothing about it. They say that if you love him, you will obey his rules. Guys believe that it's supposed to be that way. We must do things according to their way, and it will be hard to convince them otherwise.

Even though several young women and men at Masani related and adjusted to the traditional gender role expressed above, there were exceptions. A few of the black female respondents were clear about the importance of acting according to their own personal needs, and thus exercised agency outside 'pre-scripted' roles. The description below by a black female at Masani illustrates how females subverted the hegemonic script of male dominance. As she suggests, she has the ability to establish different rules and thus create a different identity:

> Girls are falling for their threats. They are so powerless and weak in putting out their ideas. They come to circumstances where they live with the decisions that their partners make for them. We have got our own responsibility too. I was born alone in this world, and I can manage by myself if a guy wants me to do something I don't want to do. Girls have to learn [to] stand ... up for themselves! They have to understand that the decision itself lies in the person. If you are strong inside, you are able to make decisions for yourself also in a relationship. Girls put their lives at risk too often to please a guy.

The scripts where women are able to reject sexual contact are not in accordance with the dominant discourse of the traditional script in the community in which Masani is located (O'Sullivan et al, 2006). As in the above, some of the girls in this school seemed confident, despite the restrictive gender roles expected of them. They could create a different reality for themselves, one that made them less susceptible to male dominance. According to Igra and Irwin (1996), such self-confidence may lead to behaviour change. An individual's challenge of the existing roles is thereby an important premise for changing the modes of sexual life in a society (Simon & Gagnon, 1987). Thus the black female respondents' challenge of the dominant gender roles privileged in their community can potentially lead to changes in the way in which women position themselves or are positioned over time.

On the other hand, at Birkenhead, women's roles appeared less prescriptive and less shaped by a hegemonic masculine discourse than at Masani. Females in this environment were more independent and also better able to make choices based on notions of equality in relationships. A white female respondent at this school described the equality of status as follows: 'For me, it's important to be equal to my partner. My opinion should count as much as his. I would not accept to be looked down upon or to feel like I owe him something.'

Another white female respondent described how negotiations in a sexual relation could develop. Her description, though, not only suggests equality of status, but also the woman's role in thinking about 'risk' and 'protection'. She said:

> In the new generation the girls are in control of the relationships most of the time. They make the decisions about sex and condoms. She is always the one who thinks about the consequences. The guy will go for what the girl says as long as he gets sex.

The ways in which men and women are socialised and the concomitant 'expected' gender roles not only shaped responses, but also produced different female subjectivities. Equality and non-discrimination between males and females were more prominent at Birkenhead, whereas at Masani, patterns of less equal power relations were evident. Males in the former environment were, more often than not, in control of relationships and seemed dominant in negotiating their nature and form. However, females tended to be more proactive and they seemed to have more control over their sexual choices. They spoke of themselves as possessing equal power in relationships.

The ability to express sexual interest in a partner was also considered important by the girls at Birkenhead. However, a parent of a female at this school was cautious and less accepting of such a practice. She recognised this as a deviation from what she saw as the traditional script where women are expected to be sexually passive, and recipients of men's sexual advances instead. She suggested that equality and females taking control in relationships are recent phenomena. She described this 'new' role by the predominantly white females in this way:

> It's changing that the boy is the only one taking the initiative. Sometimes, I see girls tend to want their way, and then they take the lead. They are more aware of their position and often the dominant part in the relationships of today. Has it to do with the women's rights and standing up for yourself? They are becoming too overpowering for me.

This parent's ambivalence is echoed in her response, as she views this as 'not the way to go'. To her, females in this position may also put themselves in sexually risky situations where their choices can lead to unintended consequences.

Both female groups expressed the ability to make sexual decisions outside of the 'expected', even though this was more common at Birkenhead. Females at Birkenhead told stories of their ability to refuse sex with a partner, decline sex without the use of a condom, demand an HIV test from a partner before engaging in a sexual relationship, end relationships where their opinions were not respected, and not give into pressure from or accept coercion or violence from a partner. And so, while it was common for the white female respondents to suggest an ability to express their personal needs and their refusal to engage in risky sexual activity, some black females also expressed similar sentiments about control over their bodies. The latter, though, were more keenly aware that this was against the dominant expectation in their community.

Thus, the gender roles in the two environments, while divergent, were both open to different possibilities, but in different ways. At Birkenhead, females, it would seem, had more choices. The gender norms and expectations here were more dynamic and were not always constructed according to the social expectations in the environment (Connell,

2000; Morrell, 2001). Both the female and male respondents at Birkenhead emphasised that it was acceptable, for example, for women to take the sexual initiative. As a result, women at Birkenhead seemed better able to construct a sexual identity independent of men, unlike their counterparts at Masani, where sexual identity was intricately linked with social expectations and hegemonic gender role identities — ones framed within a masculinised and often heterosexualised discourse.

The study's findings show that for young black females, women's sexuality was restrictive and shaped by a particular set of sociocultural norms. Women here, it would seem, are expected to display 'decent' behaviour, keep their virginity and avoid sexual contact before being involved in a serious relationship (preferably marriage). While most of the female respondents claimed that they were trying to live up to such standards, some thought differently, as the earlier discussion suggested. The sex role theory offers some explanation of this behaviour, suggesting that people under most circumstances act according to expectations in their social environment (Hargreaves, 1986), and that women and men behave differently because of different social expectations (Connell, 1987).

The social expectations, in the case of the respondents at Masani, seemed also to be underpinned by a patriarchal discourse that confirmed men's control in sexual encounters. Women's relative disempowerment with regard to men can thus be viewed as a critical factor influencing women's greater risk of infection. Interestingly, though, females at Birkenhead also seemed to be at risk, but for very different reasons. Their 'freedom' to choose partners and the ability to influence the nature of the relationship also create risks. As Giddens (1991) suggests, modernity is about risk, choice and uncertainty. It would seem, therefore, that the social expectations within the Birkenhead environment, while open and supposedly more favourable, also created risk of infection.

Masculinity and sexual identity

The concept of 'hegemonic masculinity' (Connell, 1987) emphasises that many variations of the concept of 'masculinity' exist within and among societies. This challenges the idea that gender identity is natural, unchanging and 'given'. Different communities would thus display particular forms of masculinity, and what is perceived as the most desirable and as wielding the most power — a 'hegemonic masculinity' — will differ (Connell, 1987). Privileged masculinity in the community in which Masani is located was characterised by discipline and authority in relation to a partner, which in turn gave one status among other men. These unequal gender power relations were confirmed by all the respondents at Masani, as the following quotation from a male respondent illustrates:

> It's important that she listens to me when I'm saying something. If we disagree, I have the last word. I wouldn't accept my girlfriend to do what she wants. I can explain it to her, so that she will understand that my decision is the best. The girls like that the men decide for them (Black male respondent no. 1).

Moreover, sexual practices were underpinned by meanings that associated sex with gifts, and manhood with the ability to attract and often maintain multiple sexual partners. It appeared, too, that the construction of sexuality and the attendant sexual behaviours of men in this largely Xhosa-speaking community were to a large extent based on particular understandings of manhood; conceptions that not only produced unequal power relations that disadvantaged women, but also made boys and men victims of the unequal power relations, despite the advantages offered them by society (Makahye, 2005). Such constructions of a particular masculinity that places men in a superior position detrimentally prevents them from seeking information and protecting themselves and their partners from HIV infection. A female respondent explains the construction of masculinity and the dominant male role at Masani as follows:

> Guys want to control girls, be brave and have the leadership. It's important for men to be in power. They think they are more powerful than women. Boys always say they have to have several partners because they need to satisfy their sexual needs. Some think that if they don't have sex all the time, the sperm will go up to their brain and affect their mind (Black female respondent no. 9).

At Masani, gender inequality is also, in part, evidenced by reports of participation in involuntary sexual interactions by female respondents:

> The girls aren't able to tell a boy her opinion and be heard. If she doesn't accept the boy's opinion and listens to him, he will probably hit her or leave her for another girlfriend. He will try to discourage her and make her feel useless. Most girls will then fall and say they will have sex with him even if they don't want to. She might be afraid to tell him 'no'. He has the power and will force himself on her anyway (Black female respondent no. 3).

Another female from Masani put it this way:

> Some guys are stubborn, and they will do it by force even if she doesn't want to. I think it's about masculinity. They want to push their egos. The girls might say no, but some guys wouldn't respect that. That's a common thing in the relationships in the townships. You see it every weekend. They will still stay together afterwards (Black female respondent no. 9).

The findings suggest that manhood in this community is generally associated with authority, aggression and power. These characteristics are in line with Connell's (1987) broader definition of 'hegemonic masculinity' in which sex is looked upon as men's right.

At Birkenhead, however, masculine identities were not tied up in a collective identity. The consequence for sexual identity construction was the different ways in which females understood and created a sexual identity. This illustrates how groups of the same gender give social support to and maintain men's sexual life (Laumann & Gagnon, 1995) by compliance.

Both the individuals and the institutions contributing to constructions of sexuality often reproduce, but often also challenge, the dominant notions of sexuality in a society (Simon & Gagnon, 1987; Laumann & Gagnon, 1995). Individual responses to the 'expected' and 'acceptable' scripts will vary in different contexts. What the results suggest was that the scripts that specify acceptable sexual behaviour at Birkenhead were more flexible and open to transformation, with individuals feeling better able to exercise different choices. An individual's behaviour was not always tied to a collective identity that mediated constructions of a sexual self in a restrictive manner. Individuals at Masani were much more aware of how their collective identity shaped their individual choices.

Choice for the females in this environment was more often than not mediated through a patriarchal lens that defined 'acceptable' sexual behaviour.

Sexual coercion and violence

It is estimated that one in six women in South Africa is in an abusive relationship (Walker et al, 2004). A study by Wood and Jewkes (2001) among the Xhosa in Ngangelizwe in the Eastern Cape disclosed sexual violence against women in the form of forced sex, encroachment and multiple sexual partners. Another study among Xhosa teenagers in Khayelitsha in Cape Town revealed male dominance, coercion and violence against women (Wood & Jewkes, 1997b; see also Da Cruz, 2004). There is also evidence of a connection among violence, sexual risk behaviour and reproductive health (Karim, 2005).

This study revealed that none of the respondents at Birkenhead and relatively few respondents at Masani talked about experiences with physical abuse in their relationships. None of the black male respondents reported having forced their female partners to engage in sexual activity. However, seven of the female respondents at Masani reported that on several occasions they had had involuntary (and unprotected) sex. They narrated how their male partners coerced them into taking part in certain activities, especially sex. One put it this way:

> Some boys are really controlling, and we can do nothing about it. If he wants to have sex, you got to have sex. Otherwise he will beat you up. Guys usually force girls to have sex with them. Most of them don't take no for an answer. What mostly happens is that she will fall for the threat and sleep with him. In some cases it's because of the violence you will stay with him (Black female respondent no. 2).

Involuntary and unprotected sex often originated from a feeling of pressure, force or obligation to a partner. Although Igra and Irwin (1996:35) define risk behaviour as 'those behaviours, undertaken volitionally, whose outcomes remain uncertain with the possibility of an identifiable negative health outcome', involuntary and unprotected sex as described above is often not volitional. Igra and Irwin's (1996) definition of risk behaviour ignores the factors outside a person's free will.

It was difficult to estimate the extent of coercion and violence because of the sensitivity linked to such issues. However, many of the black women told stories about other women's experiences of forced sex and rape. In this way, a gender role pattern based on hegemonic masculinity and patriarchy reproduced the notion of girls being unable to make independent choices in terms of their reproductive health. Extensive literature shows a relationship among gender violence, unequal gender power relations and risk of HIV infection (Wood & Jewkes, 1997b; LeClerc-Madlala, 2002a; Walker et al, 2004; Kauffman, 2004; Karim, 2005).

Women lose the authority to make decisions about their own bodies and health when the gender role patterns are based on convictions that women should be submissive to and controlled by men (Da Cruz, 2004; Walker et al, 2004). When the gender dynamics are characterised by men's 'right' to sex, it may lead to sexual coercion and violence (Wood & Jewkes, 1997b; 2001; LeClerc-Madlala, 2002a). LeClerc-Madlala (2002a) argues for a discussion on the prevailing acceptance of sexual violence against women as 'normal' sexual behaviour, men's right to control sexual encounters, and thus women's disadvantageous position in negotiations related to sex and the use of condoms. In the last demographic and health survey in South Africa, 13% of the women reported having being beaten by a partner (Karim, 2005). To negotiate safe sex and protection under circumstances where women face physical violence is often impossible.

Stigmatising attitudes and the feeling of being at risk

The white respondents consistently stereotyped those they considered at risk of HIV infection. Black skin colour was the main point of reference to infection. In doing so, they distanced themselves from the possibility of personal risk. The data showed that the white youth imagined a sense of immunity to HIV infection based on ethnicity, irrespective of their educational background and specific knowledge about HIV/AIDS:

> Some white people think they are immune to HIV infection. They consider the African people to be beneath them. Mostly there are the black South Africans dying from AIDS. White people don't realise that a lot of white people are also infected. They tell themselves that it only exists with the African people and in the townships. Black people are looked upon as the dirty race or the impure or stupid. We have learned about the differences in cultures in class. We learn that most of the non-whites are uneducated about AIDS. That's why we are less vulnerable (White female respondent no. 5).

The respondents at Birkenhead viewed sexual behaviour as a personal choice and claimed that AIDS was caused by carelessness. These respondents' statements describe behaviour as something exclusively based on personal choice. This ignores the complex interrelationship between the individual and the social factors associated with gender and power (Wood & Jewkes, 1997b; 2001), which are often obstacles in situations where there are unequal gender power relations and where sexual decision making is the domain of the male (Da Cruz, 2004).

According to what the white respondents believe, HIV/AIDS infection follows ethnic lines in South Africa (Breidlid, 2005; Gouws & Karim, 2005). Thus, existing prejudices based on race and ethnicity encouraged stigma and discrimination associated with HIV (Gouws & Karim, 2005). Many of the white respondents argued that HIV infection mostly arose from black people's cultural beliefs and practices, such as polygamy. They also associated female subordination and male promiscuity with black people. If such characteristics indicate vulnerability to HIV infection, it may explain why the white adolescents perceive themselves as immune to HIV infection.

The white respondents in this study did not think they were in danger of contracting HIV through sexual contact. They were more concerned with possible infection through medical treatment, blood transfusion, wounds and rape. They also did not view their sexual behaviour as something that placed them at risk of infection. HIV/AIDS was a pandemic of the other, of which they were not a part. These respondents ignored elements such as alcohol and drug use, which may lead to sexually risky behaviour and consequently put them at risk of infection.

The stereotypes about black people often function as an emotional and social protection and reduce the white adolescents' feeling of being at risk, but notions of invincibility and invulnerability to infection could lead to sexual behaviour that is HIV predisposing among this group. Overall, the tendency to blame the HIV problem on 'others' may lead to individuals' feeling less responsible for their own actions. By indirectly placing the possibilities for change outside the individuals' authority, a distance from the HIV/AIDS challenge is produced. The phenomenon of distancing oneself from the disease may have tremendous consequences for adolescents' sexual behaviour and the use of contraceptives, especially at Birkenhead.

Alcohol and drug use and sexual risk behaviour

Peer pressure, a modern gender role pattern and stigmatising beliefs may be identified as responsible for the sexual risk behaviour among adolescents at Birkenhead. In addition, the use of alcohol and drugs was also strongly linked with risky sexual behaviour at Birkenhead. From the data collected at Masani, there seemed to be less of a connection between intoxication and sexual behaviour.

At Birkenhead there was an understanding among the respondents that alcohol and drug use reduced sexual restraint. Among this group, normally unacceptable sexual behaviour was explained as an effect of intoxication. Several of the respondents talked about sensational sexual behaviour by both genders where attention from peers was seen as very important. The respondents considered alcohol and drug use as interlinked with a range of sexual behaviours that also had serious emotional and health-related consequences. This applied to quickly established and rapidly changing sexual relations, early sexual debut, multiple partners and unprotected sex. As DiClemente and Cobb (1999) suggest, participating in one kind of risk behaviour seems to increase the chance of other risky activities.

Discussion

'Open' and 'closed' scripts

Individuals learn the scripts for sexual behaviour in environments in which they make meaning of their lives. According to Simon and Gagnon (1987), sexuality is acquired through learning processes in which the individual learns scripts for sexual behaviour in accordance with what is acceptable in specific localities. Sexual acts, sexual desire and 'living out' sexuality achieve a meaning when they are ascribed certain qualities and content by the social and cultural context (Gagnon & Simon, 2005). Individual choices are thus a result of interaction between the individuals' wishes and desires, and the social and cultural practices in which the person is socialised (Laumann & Gagnon, 1995). This interrelationship is complex. Often individuals comply and reproduce the dominant discourse, thus producing what I refer to as a 'closed' sexual script. A closed script, in this chapter, is characterised by sexual cultural practices based on a patriarchal discourse, gender inequality, sexual violence, multiple sexual partners among men, negative attitudes towards condom use, fatalistic attitudes and myths based on magic and supernatural explanations, and pressures to prove fertility (LeClerc-Madlala, 2002a). According to LeClerc-Madlala (2002a), these factors contribute to a high-risk environment, especially for women. High levels of awareness and knowledge about reproductive health are undermined by such cultural norms and values and thus make individual choices and sexual negotiation difficult. Generally, both women and men at Masani tended to comply with the dominant social and cultural practices. Answers like 'that's just the way it is' from some of the female informants at Masani when explaining the prevailing gender inequality illustrate this point. Thus, men were not alone in maintaining and reproducing the asymmetric gender role patterns; women were complicit in their reproduction.

Those who act differently, as some females from Masani illustrate, were fully aware of the consequences of doing so. Thus, even in circumstances characterised by a 'closed' script, where gender roles are less fluid and where patriarchy and a 'hegemonic masculinity' define acceptable sexualities, some individual females still exercised the choice to act outside the 'prescribed' behaviour. These females were aware of how the social and cultural practices of the community and adherence to a collective identity not only established, but also reproduced and maintained male dominance and gender inequality.

The consequences of the above are great when understood in a context where the risk of sexually transmitted diseases and HIV infection is high. The perceived invulnerability associated with the male role is fertile ground for sexually risky behaviour that includes, among others, a lack of condom use and multiple sexual partners (Karim, 2005). These behaviours create women's vulnerability to HIV infection within the existing gender dynamics. The challenge communities such as the one above face is to develop strategies that foster change in gender roles without undermining male security and identity (Makahye, 2005).

The variation in gender role expectations at Birkenhead offered females many more options in constructing sexual identities that did not always adhere to those dominant in the school or community. They also seemed better able to articulate their choices — ones that were independent of the collective or dominant practice. This flexibility in the relation between the individual and the collective I refer to as an 'open' script. Such a script privileges the individual over the collective and offers women a more active role in determining their sexual choices and positioning.

What is striking, though, is that in both open and closed scripts, women's roles and the sexual decisions they make cannot be extricated from those of males.

Conclusion

As the chapter has shown, the reasons behind sexually risky behaviour are complex and require a nuanced reading of the social landscape; one that includes, but also extends beyond, the categories of race and ethnicity. What the findings show, however, is a difference in how communities with closed scripts respond to the pandemic compared to those who subscribe to a more open script. It is obvious that the closed script offers fewer opportunities for transformation, making it essential that intervention programmes incorporate strategies that begin to engage with the challenges that a closed script produces.

Individual choices and decisions are often mediated through a host of social and cultural norms and practices, even in the light of imminent risk. In communities where an open script is more prevalent, there is evidence that it sometimes opens up avenues that are also clearly detrimental to the struggle against the pandemic. In such communities, the feelings of 'invincibility' and 'immunity' to the disease also result in risky behaviour, not the least linked to alcohol and drugs.

Ultimately, intervention strategies that do not account for how meaning is mediated through a complex set of discourses and contexts often 'miss the mark' and offer costly solutions with little effect.

PART 4

HIV/AIDS EDUCATIONAL RESEARCH:

EPISTEMOLOGICAL AND METHODOLOGICAL IMPLICATIONS

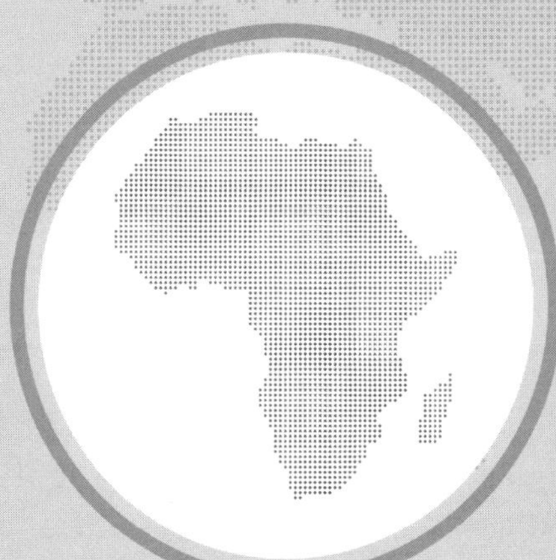

SUB-SAHARAN AFRICA

Chapter 10

Jean Baxen
University of Cape Town

Anders Breidlid
Oslo University College

Afterword: Towards a Hermeneutic Understanding of HIV/AIDS in South Africa

Introduction

The AIDS pandemic is threatening the democratic foundation of the new South Africa. As Steinberg (2008:6) states, 'a new democracy is an era of resurging life', but in this case the consequences might be far-reaching. There is recognition that the struggle against HIV/AIDS is still in its infancy, with some interpretations not helping to deal with the problem.

Responses and interpretations of the pandemic are often expressed in ways that do not always offer choice to, especially, the more vulnerable members of the population – women and youth. In this book, the experiences, attitudes and opinions of youth and young children, teachers, religious leaders and ordinary people are recounted, providing a portrait of the complexity of the problem and illustrating how it finds expression across discursive spaces. The book tells different stories, contradictory stories and controversial stories; stories told both by South Africans and Norwegians. Importantly, though, all the contributors share one vision: to use this book as a vehicle to combat a disease that is about to undermine the growth and prosperity of a fledgling democracy and rainbow nation.

This afterword brings together two main themes emerging as key aspects that need iteration. First, it focuses on government responses and second on the dominant discourses that ought to be accounted for in any future responses and interventions.

South African government responses to HIV/AIDS: Challenges and issues

The effect of the pandemic on the social and economic landscape of South Africa is well documented. Where six million people (out of a population of 46 million) are HIV-positive, where life expectancy has dropped to 52 years, where more than half of all public hospital admissions are AIDS related and more than a quarter of the national health budget is going to fighting the disease, this country cannot afford ineffective and inefficient strategies and responses.

The impact of HIV/AIDS on the education system has not only been the focus of much conjecture, but also numerous studies, as chapters in this book have illustrated. Its devastating effect on the education system and on learners and teachers has become more visible with studies like those by the Human Science Research Council (eg Peltzer et al, 2005; Simbayi et al, 2005).

Leaders in the country, in particular the former state president, Thabo Mbeki, and the former health minister, Manto Tshabalala-Msimang, have not been helpful in shaping peoples' responses to the pandemic. Both politicians offered not only controversial, but also unconventional and questionable scientific alternatives. The result has been a population ravaged by the pandemic, yet still confused and receiving mixed messages from its leaders. South Africa is a nation that at one level is perplexed about the disease's social and material impact and on another level is ambivalent in its beliefs, attitudes, and subsequent responses and actions regarding the disease. It is little wonder that literature on HIV/AIDS that focuses on the critical issues of violence, stigma, social and cultural practices and their intersection with discourses on gender, sexuality and disease has only emerged in the last few years.

The Mbeki government's denialist position has negatively affected everyday conceptions of the pandemic, fueling responses that have made behaviour change slow, even in the face of adequate knowledge. In addition, government's response, which targets education as a key strategy in responding to the pandemic, has, for the most part, used a medical discourse that assumes (a) linearity and positive correlation between knowledge and behaviour; and (b) a decontextualised body that operates outside a context marked by a complex array of intersecting discourses. Such assumptions have led to the development and implementation of a host of interventions, many of which offered more knowledge about protection, treatment and care, but have not gone far enough in asking questions about where, discursively, this knowledge is mediated. The consequence has been one-size-fits-all modernist interventions that provide 'more' knowledge. They overlook (a) deeper epistemological concerns about the frames of references used to interpret and mediate this knowledge, and (b) deeply politicised, raced, classed, gendered, sexualised and patriarchal social spaces within which individuals and collectives make meaning of their lives. The social and cultural practices that act as the mediatory filters used by many people to understand themselves in relation to the pandemic (and which are potentially still great barriers to behaviour change) have often been left unattended in intervention programmes.

The time has come to insert a new discourse into programmes about HIV/AIDS; one whose epistemology is rooted outside positivist orientations that assume an easy correspondence between knowledge and behaviour. Change agents (government, donors and organisations) represent the groups that possess knowledge and experience of how the disease is to be fought, whereas the population has knowledge that is not always transformed into healthier practice. The challenge thus arises of how to offer information in a way that addresses the relevant social and cultural practices without alienating communities.

The new health minister, Barbara Hogan, has indicated a radical change in the authorities' attitudes towards HIV/AIDS in general and its treatment and care; in particular, acknowledging that the government's policies over the past ten years failed in offering informed directives. She has promised to step up the fight against HIV/AIDS, appealing also to the scientific community to come up with better tools to fight the disease. In describing the change in attitude by the new minister, one commentator put it this way: 'Health has been rescued from the madness of lemons, garlic and beetroot, which are now restored to their role as nutritious fruit and vegetables, liberated from being the weapons of mass destruction that Manto [Tshabalala-Msimang, the previous health minister] had made them (*Mail & Guardian Online*, 2008)'. While these new policies of the government are welcome, the situation will not change overnight.

Taking account of mediatory discourses: Towards more effective interventions

Sex is the most life-giving of activities: 'That a new nation's citizens are dying from sex seems to be an attack on ordinary people's and a nation's generative capacities, an insult too ghastly to stomach' (Steinberg, 2008:6). The medical fact that the disease is most pervasively spread through sexual contact (and mostly prevalent among heterosexual populations) requires responses that take account of (a) how discourses of disease and sexuality shape and mediate everyday responses to the pandemic; (b) the discursive nature of the disease; (c) ways in which meaning making is mediated by and through particular social and cultural practices; and (d) the contextual embeddedness of the pandemic.

Sexuality is at the core of our being — the most natural thing about us — yet it is also the most difficult to explain (Weeks in Phillips & Reay, 2002). As a phenomenon that touches the heart of who we are, it often works as a producing and interpretive script from and through which social, political and moral acts are read and sometimes produced and reproduced (Baxen, 2006:103). Although many societies over time have tried to restrict sexual behaviour through a host of regulatory mechanisms, restraining it has been a challenge. Understood from this perspective, it is not surprising that HIV/AIDS is much more than a disease that simply *infects* the body; it is a symbolic bearer of a host of meanings (Baxen, 2006). It invokes aspects of our identities and is as much about sexuality, morality, politics, social marginality, dominance and power as it is a disease. Any investigation into HIV/AIDS, therefore, has to consider its associations with the broader discourses of sexuality and disease.

The way societies make meaning of their sexual lives is not easily accepted, and all kinds of mystical explanations are sometimes given to explain the occurrences of diseases such as HIV/AIDS. Steinberg (2008:15), for example, explains that people with certain cultural practices sometimes think as follows: '[S]ome people have maybe sent a demon to have sex with me: a demon with HIV. That is why I am scared to test. I think I will test positively'. In other instances, people refrain from being tested for fear of being stigmatised and even sometimes ostracised, particularly in the rural villages where individual identities are intricately mediated through a collective identity and membership in particular social and cultural practices, which make it difficult for an individual to exercise choice without serious negative consequences. As Steinberg (2008:6) says: 'Where there is AIDS, there is blame. It is said in the villages that the virus was hatched in laboratories to be let loose on blacks until whites become an electoral majority'. And since people are scared of being tested, they do not access antiretroviral drugs that might improve their life situation substantially. The result is that people are dying a few metres from access to medication that could potentially save their lives.

Importantly too, the changing nature of the pandemic necessitates responses that take account of aspects such as those discussed in this book; ones not easily accessible if the epistemological and methodological orientations remain those that are embedded in exclusively Western frames of references, on the one hand, and socially disembedded contexts, on the other.

Bibliography

Abdul-Wahhab, M M. 2001. 'Islam.' In R. A. Smith (ed.). *Encyclopedia of AIDS: A Social, Political, Cultural, and Scientific Record of the HIV Epidemic*, pp. 391–93. New York: Penguin.

Abt Associates. 2001. *The Impending Catastrophe Revisited*. Commissioned report. Johannesburg: loveLife/Henry J. Kaiser Family Foundation.

Agrawal, H K, Roa, R S P, Chandrashekar, S & Coulter, J B S. 1999. 'Knowledge of and attitudes to HIV/AIDS of senior secondary school pupils and trainee teachers in Udupi District, Karnataka, India.' *Annals of Tropical Paediatrics: International Child Health*, vol. 19, no. 2. pp. 143–49.

Ahlberg, B M. 1994. 'Is there a distinct African sexuality? A critical response to Caldwell.' *Africa*, vol. 64, no. 2. pp. 221–42.

Ahmed, A K. 1999. 'The impact of HIV/AIDS on the Muslim community in the Western Cape: A critical analysis of Muslim responses to the AIDS pandemic.' Unpublished thesis, Department of Religious Studies, University of Cape Town.

Akoulouze, R, Rugalema, G & Khanye, V. 2001. *Taking Stock of Promising Approaches in HIV/AIDS and Education in Sub-Saharan Africa: What Works, Why and How.* <http://wwwadeanet.org>. Accessed 20 February 2003.

Allen, P L. 2000. *The Wages of Sin: Sex and Disease, Past and Present*. Chicago & London: University of Chicago Press.

Allen, P L. 2001. *Disease and History: Must the Past be Prologue?* <http://www.thebody.com/content/whatis/art30989.html>. Accessed 15 December 2008.

Allen-Meares, P & Shapiro, C H. (eds). 1989. *Adolescent Sexuality: New Challenges for Social Work.* New York: Haworth Press.

Allott, R. 1999. *Religion and Science — Sex and Society: Forms and Processes of Cohesion*. <http://cogprints.org/3159/01/cohesion.htm>. Accessed 30 March 2006.

Archie-Booker, D E, Cervero, R M & Langone, C A. 1999. 'The politics of planning culturally relevant AIDS prevention education for African-American women.' *Adult Education Quarterly,* vol. 49, no. 4. pp. 163–76.

AVERT. 2007. *AVERT South Africa HIV & AIDS Statistics*. <http://www.avert.org/safricastats.htm>. Accessed 15 February 2007.

Babbie, E. 1999. *The Basics of Social Research.* Belmont: Wadsworth.

Babbie, E & Mouton, J, Vorster, P & Prozesky, B. 2001. *The Practice of Social Research*. Cape Town: Oxford University Press.

Bankole, A. 2004. *Risk and Protection: Youth and HIV/AIDS in Sub-Saharan Africa*. New York: Alan Guttmacher Institute.

Barnett, T & Whiteside, A. 2002. *AIDS in the Twenty-First Century: Disease and Globalization*. Basingstoke: Palgrave Macmillan.

Baxen, J. 2005. 'HIV/AIDS educational research: Beyond more of the same to asking different epistemological questions.' *UWC Papers in Education*, vol. 3. pp. 58–63.

Baxen, J. 2006. 'An analysis of the factors shaping teachers' understanding of HIV/AIDS.' Unpublished doctoral thesis, University of Cape Town.

Baxen, J. 2008. 'Using narratives to develop a hermeneutic understanding of HIV/AIDS in South Africa.' *Compare: Journal of Comparative Education*, vol. 38, no. 3. pp. 307–19.

Baxen, J & Breidlid, A. 2004. 'Researching HIV/AIDS and education in sub-Saharan Africa: Examining the gaps and challenges.' *Journal of Education*, vol. 34. pp. 9–29.

Bennel, P. 2003. 'Telling it how it is? The UNAIDS 2003 update on the AIDS epidemic in Sub-Saharan Africa.' Mimeo.

Berger, P L. 1977. *Facing up to Modernity*. New York: Basic Books.

Berndt, T J. 1996. 'Transitions in friendship and friends' influence.' In J. A. Graber et al (eds). *Transitions through Adolescence: Interpersonal Domains and Context*, pp. 57–83. Mahwah: Lawrence Erlbaum.

Binsbergen, W. 2003. *Challenges for the Sociology of Religion in the African Context*. Rotterdam: African Studies Centre, Faculty of Philosophy, Erasmus University.

Bourdieu, P. 1976. 'Systems of education and systems of thought.' In R Dale, G Esland & M. McDonald (eds). *Schooling and Capitalism: A Sociological Reader*. London: Routledge & Kegan Paul.

Bourdieu, P. 1990. *The Logic of Practice*. Stanford: Stanford University Press.

Bourdieu, P. 1993. *Sociology in Question*. London: Sage.

Bourdieu, P & Passeron, J. 1977. *Reproduction in Education, Society and Culture.* London: Sage.

Bradshaw, D, Nannan, N, Laubscher, L, Groenewald, P, Joubert, J, Nojilana, B, Norman, R, Pieterse, D, & Schneider, M. 2004. *South African National Burden of Disease Study 2000: Estimates of Provincial Mortality.* Cape Town: Medical Research Council.

Breakwell, G M. (ed.). 1992. *Social Psychology of Identity and Self-concept*. London: Academic Press.

Breidlid, A. 2002. 'Schooling, tradition and modernity in South Africa.' *UWC Papers in Education*, 2, December: pp. 37–50.

Breidlid, A. 2005. 'HIV/AIDS, cultural constraints and education.' *UWC Papers in Education,* 6(3): 50–57.

Bronfenbrenner, U. 1979. *The Ecology of Human Development: Experiments by Nature and Design.* Cambridge, Mass.: Harvard University Press.

Buczekiewicz, M. & Carnegie, R. 2001. 'The Ugandan Life Skills Initiative.' *Health Education*, vol. 101, no. 1. pp. 15–21.

Bullough, V L & Bullough, B. 1994. *Human Sexuality: An Encyclopedia*. New York & London: Garland.

Burman, E. 1994. *Deconstructing Developmental Psychology*. New York: Routledge.

Butler, J P. 1990. *Gender Trouble: Feminism and the Subversion of Identity*. New York: Routledge.

Butler, J P. 1993. *Bodies that Matter*. New York: Routledge.

Caldwell, J C. 1999. *Rethinking the African AIDS Epidemic*. <http://www.arha.org.au/papersandarticles/OP%202.pdf>. Accessed 10 October 2008.

Caldwell, J C, Caldwell, P & Quiggin, P. 1989. 'The social context of AIDS in sub-Saharan Africa.' *Population and Development Review*, vol. 15, no. 2. pp. 185–233.

Campbell, C. 2003. *'Letting Them Die': Why HIV/AIDS Prevention Programmes Fail.* Oxford: International African Institute in association with James Currey.

Campbell, C & Mzaidume, Z. 2001. 'Grassroots participation, peer education, and HIV prevention by sex workers in South Africa.' *American Journal of Public Health*, 91(12): 1978–86.

Cashmore, E. 2004. *Encyclopedia of Race and Ethnic Studies.* London: Routledge.

Chirambo, K. 2008. *The Political Cost of AIDS in Africa: Evidence from Six Countries.* Pretoria: Idasa.

Claire, M R & Lee, R M. (eds). 1993. *Researching Sensitive Topics*. Newbury: Sage.

Cohen, D. 2002. 'HIV and education in sub-Saharan Africa: Responding to the impact.' *Perspectives in Education,* vol. 20, no. 2. pp. 13–23.

Cole, M & Cole, S. 2001. *The Development of Children.* New York: Worth.

Coleman, J & Roker, D. 1998. *Teenage Sexuality: Health, Risk and Education*. Amsterdam: Hardwood Academic.

Connell, R W. 1987. *Gender and Power: Society, the Person and Sexual Politics.* Cambridge: Polity Press.

Connell, R W. 1996. *Maskuliniteter.* Gõteborg: Daidalos AB.

Connell, R W. 2000: *The Men and the Boys.* Cambridge: Polity Press.

Coombe, C. 2000a. *Managing the Impact of HIV/AIDS on the Education Sector*. Pretoria: C:\cec\HIV\South Africa\FINALECAHIV.doc.

Coombe, C. 2000b. 'Keeping the education system healthy: Managing the impact of HIV/AIDS on education in South Africa.' *Current issues in Comparative Education*, vol. 3, no. 1. pp. 14–27.

Coombe, C. 2001. HIV and Education. Pretoria: C: My Documents\AAAPAPERS\CONSTRUCTMAIN.doc.

Coombe, C & Kelly, M J. 2001. 'Education as a vehicle for combating HIV/AIDS.' *Prospects Quarterly Review of Education*, vol. 31, no. 3. pp. 435–43.

Cornwall, A & Lindisfarne, N. 1994. 'Dislocating masculinity: Gender, power and anthropology.' In A. Cornwall & N. Lindisfarne (eds). *Dislocating Masculinities: Comparative Ethnographies.* London: Routledge.

Corsaro, W. 1997. *The Sociology of Childhood*. California: Pine Forge Press.

Cosman, C. 2001. *The Elementary Forms of Religious Life.* Oxford & New York: Oxford University Press.

Cousins, M & Hussain, A. 1985. *Michael Foucault*. Hong Kong: Macmillan.

Crewe, M. 2002. 'Reflections on the South African HIV/AIDS epidemic.' *Society in Transition*, vol. 33, no. 3. pp. 446–54.

Crockett, L. J. & Crouter, A. C. 1995. *Pathways through Adolescence: Individual Development in Relation to Social Contexts*. Hillsdale: L. Erlbaum.

Crossley, N. 2001. *The Social Body: Habit, Identity and Desire*. London: Sage.

Da Cruz, C C B R. 2004. 'From policy to practice: The anthropology of condom use.' In K D Kauffman & D. Lindauer (eds). *AIDS and South Africa: The Social Expression of a Pandemic*, pp. 136–60. New York: Palgrave Macmillan.

Dalin, P, Rolff, H & Kleekam, B. 1993. *Changing the School Culture.* London: Cassell IMTEC Foundation.

Damen, L. 1987. *Culture Learning: The Fifth Dimension in the Language Classroom.* Reading, Mass.: Addison-West. <http://www.carla.umn.edu/culture/definitions.html>. Accessed 5 May 2005.

Darnell, F & Höem, A. 1996. *Taken to Extremes: Education in the Far North.* Oslo: Scandinavian University Press.

DeLamater, J. 1987. 'A sociological approach.' In J. Geer & W. T. O'Donohue (eds). *Theories of Human Sexuality: Perspectives in Sexuality: Behaviour, Research and Therapy*, pp. 237–56. New York & London: Plenum Press.

De la Rey, C. 1999. 'Career narratives of women professors in South Africa.' Unpublished doctoral thesis, University of Cape Town.

Denzin, N K & Lincoln, S. 1998. *Collecting and Interpreting Qualitative Materials.* London: Sage.

DiClemente, R J. (ed.). 1992. *Adolescents and AIDS: A Generation in Jeopardy*. Newbury Park: Sage.

DiClemente, R J & Cobb, B. 1999. 'Adolescent health promotion and disease prevention.' In J. M. Raczynski & R J DiClemente (eds). *Handbook of Health Promotion and Disease Prevention,* pp. 491–520. New York: Kluwer Academic/Plenum.

Dilley, R. 1999. *The Problem of Context*. New York: Berghahn Books.

DoE (Department of Education). 1999. *National Policy on HIV/AIDS for Learners and Educators in Public Schools*. Pretoria: Government Printer. 10 August. <http://education.pwv.gov.za/1999>.

DoE (Department of Education). 2000/02. *The HIV/AIDS Emergency: Guidelines for Educators*. Pretoria: Government Printer. <http://education.pwv.gov.za/content/documents/70.pdf>. Accessed 17 December 2004.

DoE (Department of Education). 2003a. *Develop an HIV & AIDS Plan for Your School: A Guide for School Governing Bodies and Management Teams.* Pretoria: DoE.

DoE (Department of Education). 2003b. Department of Education, 2002. *Revised National Curriculum Statement Grades R–9 (Schools): Tirisano*. Pretoria: DoE. <http://www.education.gov.za>. Accessed 10 August 2006.

DoH (Department of Health). 2007. *The HIV/AIDS and Sexually Transmitted Infection (STI) Strategic Plan for South Africa (NSP 2007–2011).* 14 March. <http://www.doh.gov.za/docs/misc/stratplan-f.html>. Accessed 10 June 2008.

Dorrington, R, Bradshaw, D, Johnson, L & Budlender, D. 2004. *The Demographic Impact of HIV/AIDS in South Africa: National Indicators for 2004*. Cape Town: Centre for Actuarial Research, University of Cape Town.

Durkheim, E. 1952. *Suicide: A Study in Sociology*. Translated by John A. Spaulding & George Simpson. New York: Free Press.

Durkheim, E. 2001. *The Elementary Forms of Religious Life.* Translated by Carol Cosman. Oxford & New York: Oxford University Press.

Easton, D E. 1999. 'Reckoning with "the sickness": Perceptions of AIDS risk and risk-reduction strategies among Puerto Rican adolescents who know PHAs.' *Anthropology and Medicine*, vol. 6, no. 1. pp. 133–42.

Education Labour Relations Council. 2005a. *Educator Attrition and Mortality in South Africa Fact-sheet.* Mobile Task Team. Pretoria: Education Labour Relations Council.

Education Labour Relations Council. 2005b. *Educator Supply and Demand in the South African Public Education System: Integrated Report.* Cape Town: Human Sciences Research Council Press.

Epstein, D & Johnson, R. 1998. *Schooling Sexualities*. Buckingham: Open University Press.

Epstein, H. 2007. *The Invisible Cure: Africa, the West, and the Fight against AIDS*. New York: Farrar, Straus & Giroux.

Erikson, E. 1968. *Identity: Youth and Crisis*. London: Faber & Faber.

Evans-Pritchard, E E. 1965. *The Position of Women in Primitive Societies and Other Essays in Social Anthropology.* London: Faber.

Fleisch, B D. 1995. 'The teachers college club: American educational discourse and the origins of Bantu education in South Africa, 1914–1951.' Doctoral thesis, Columbia University.

Friedland, R, Jankelowitz, M, De Beer, S, De Klerk, V, Khoury, T, Csizmadia, G, Paydayachee, G. & Levy, S. 1991. 'Perceptions and knowledge about the acquired immunodeficiency syndrome among students in university residences.' *South African Medical Journal*, vol. 79. pp. 149–54.

Frohlich, J. 2005. 'The impact of AIDS on the community.' In S. S. A Karim & Q. A. Karim (eds). *HIV/AIDS in South Africa*, pp. 351–70. Cambridge: Cambridge University Press.

Gacoin, A. 2006. *HIV/AIDS and Adolescents*. <http://www.aidsportal.org/Article_Details.aspx?ID=635>. Accessed 5 June 2008.

Gagnon, J. H. & Parker, R. G. 1995. 'Conceiving sexuality.' In R. G. Parker & J. H. Gagnon (eds). *Conceiving Sexuality: Approaches to Sex Research in a Postmodern World*, pp. 3–18. New York & London: Routledge.

Gagnon, J. H. & Simon, W. 2005. *Sexual Conduct: The Social Sources of Human Sexuality.* 2nd ed. New Brunswick & London: Aldine Transaction.

Gallant, M. & Maticka-Tyndale, E. 2003. 'School-based HIV prevention programmes for African youth.' *Social Science and Medicine*, vol. 58, no. 7. pp. 1337–51.

Garner, R. C. 2000. 'Safe sects? Dynamic religion and AIDS in South Africa.' *Journal of Modern African Studies*, vol. 38, no. 1. pp. 41–69.

Giddens, A. 1987. *Social Theory and Modern Sociology.* Cambridge: Polity Press.

Giddens, A. 1991. *Modernity and Self-identity: Self and Society in the Late Modern Age.* Stanford: Stanford University Press.

Giroux, A. 1981. *Ideology, Culture and the Process of Schooling.* London: Falmer Press.

Goodwin, W & Goodwin, L. 1996. *Understanding Quantitative and Qualitative Research in Early Childhood Education.* New York: Teachers College Press.

Goss, R. 2001. 'Protestant churches.' In R. A. Smith (ed.). *Encyclopedia of AIDS: A Social, Political, Cultural, and Scientific Record of the HIV Epidemic*, pp. 543–47. New York: Penguin.

Gouws, E & Karim, Q A. 2005. 'HIV infection in South Africa: The evolving epidemic.' In S. S. A Karim & Q. A. Karim (eds). *HIV/AIDS in South Africa*, pp. 48–66. Cambridge: Cambridge University Press.

Greig, A D & Taylor, J. 1999. *Doing Research with Children*. London: Sage.

Grunseit, A C & Aggleton, P. 1998. 'Lessons learned: An update on the published literature concerning the impact of HIV and sexuality education for young people.' *Health Education*, vol. 98, no. 2. pp. 45–54.

Hall, S. 1990. 'Cultural identity and diaspora.' In J. Rutherford (ed.). *Identity*. London: Lawrence & Wishart.

Hall, S & Du Gay, P. (eds). 1996. *Questions of Cultural Identity*. London: Sage.

Hargreaves, D J. 1986. 'Psychological theories of sex-role stereotyping.' In D. J. Hargreaves & A. M. Colley (eds). *The Psychology of Sex Roles*. London: Harper & Row.

Harrison, A. 2005. 'Young people and HIV/AIDS in South Africa: Prevalence of infection, risk factors and social context.' In S. S. A. Karim & Q. A. Karim (eds). *HIV/AIDS in South Africa*, pp. 262–84. Cambridge: Cambridge University Press.

Harrison, A, Xaba, N, Kunene, P. & Ntuli, N. 2001. 'Understanding young women's risk for HIV/AIDS: Adolescent sexuality and vulnerability in rural KwaZulu/Natal.' *Society in Transition*, vol. 32, no. 1. pp. 69–78.

Hartell, C. 2001. *The Status of HIV/AIDS and Education Research in South Africa*. Unpublished report. Pretoria: Faculty of Education, University of Pretoria.

Hewson, M G. 1998. 'Traditional healers in Southern Africa.' *Annals of International Medicine*, vol. 128, no. 12. pp. 1029–34.

Hickey, A. 2002. 'HIV/AIDS spending policy and intergovernmental fiscal relations.' *South African Journal of Economics*, vol. 70, no. 7. pp. 597–605.

Hofstede, G. 1984. 'National cultures and corporate cultures.' In L. A. Samovar & R. E. Porter (eds). *Communication between Cultures*. Belmont: Wadsworth.

Hogg, M & Abrams, D. 1988. *Social Identifications: A Social Psychology of Inter-group Relations and Group Processes*. London: Routledge.

HSRC (Human Sciences Research Council). 2005. *HSRC Household Survey 2005*. Cape Town: HSRC Press. <http://www.hsrc.ac.za/Media_Release-256.phtml>. Accessed 10 June 2008.

Igra, V & Irwin, C E. 1996. 'Theories of adolescent risk-taking behavior.' In R. J. DiClemente et al (eds). *Handbook of Adolescent Health Risk Behavior*, pp. 35–52. New York & London: Plenum Press.

Iverson Software. 2005. *Modern Community*. <http://www.webref.org/sociology/m/modern_community.htm%20%20%5b2006,March>. Accessed 30 March 2006.

James, A, Jenks, C & Prout, A. 1998. *Theorizing Childhood*. Cambridge: Polity Press.

Jenks, C. 1996. 'The postmodern child.' In J. Brannen & M. O. Brien (eds). *Children in Families: Research and Policy*, pp. 13–22. London: Falmer Press.

Jessor, R. (ed.). 1998. *New Perspectives on Adolescent Risk Behaviour*. Cambridge: Cambridge University Press.

Jewkes, R, Levin, J, Mbananga, N & Bradshaw, D. 2002. 'Rape of girls in South Africa.' *Lancet*, 359(9303), 26 January: 319–20. <http://www.scienceblog.com/community/older/2002/E/20023369.html>. Accessed 10 October 2008.

Johnson, S. 2000. 'The impact of AIDS on the education sector in South Africa.' Presentation at the IIEP meeting on the impact of HIV/AIDS on education. Paris, September.

Kaaya, S G, Mukoma, W, Flisher, A J & Knut-Inge K. 2002. 'School-based sexual health initiatives in Sub-Saharan Africa: A review.' *Social Dynamics*, 28(1): 64–88.

Kalichman, S C, Simbayi, L C, Kaufman, M, Cain, D, Cherry, C, Jooste, S & Mathiti, V. 2005. 'Gender attitudes, sexual violence, and HIV/AIDS risks among men and women in Cape Town, South Africa.' *Journal of Sex Research,* vol. 42, no. 4. pp. 299–305.

Karim, Q A. 2005. 'Heterosexual transmission of HIV: The importance of a gendered perspective in HIV prevention.' In S. S. A. Karim & Q. A. Karim (eds). *HIV/AIDS in South Africa*, pp. 243–61. Cambridge: Cambridge University Press.

Kaufman, C E & Stavros, S E. 2002. *'Bus Fare, Please': The Economics of Sex and Gifts among Adolescents in Urban South Africa.* Population Council. <http://www.popcouncil.org/pdfs/wp/166.pdf>. Accessed 27 January 2003.

Kauffman, K D. 2004. 'Why is South Africa the HIV capital of the world? An institutional analysis of the spread of a virus.' In K. D. Kauffman & D. L. Lindauer (eds). *AIDS and South Africa: The Social Expression of a Pandemic,* pp. 17–30. New York: Palgrave Macmillan.

Kelly, K. 2000. *Communicating for Action: A Contextual Evaluation of Youth Responses to HIV/AIDS.* Sentinel Site Monitoring and Evaluation Project report. Pretoria: Department of Health.

Kelly, K & Ntlabati, P. 2002. 'Early adolescent sex in South Africa: HIV intervention challenges.' *Social Dynamics,* vol. 28, no. 1. pp. 42–63.

Kelly, K, Ntlabati, P, Oyosi, S, Van der Riet, M & Parker, W. 2002. *Making HIV/AIDS Our Problem: Young People and the Development Challenge in South Africa*. Johannesburg: Centre for AIDS Development Research and Evaluation.

Kelly, K & Parker, W. 2000. *Communities of Practice: Contextual Mediators of Youth Response to HIV/AIDS.* Beyond Awareness Campaign report. Pretoria: Department of Health.

Kelly, M. 2002. 'Preventing HIV transmission through education.' *Perspectives in Education*, vol. 20, no. 2. pp. 1–12.

Kelly, M J. 2000. *Planning for Education in the Context of HIV/AIDS*. Paris: UNESCO/International Institute for Educational Planning.

King, R. 1999. *Sexual Behavioural Change for HIV: Where Have the Theories Taken Us?* Geneva: UNAIDS.

Krige, E J. 1968. 'Girls' puberty songs and their relation to fertility, health, morality and religion among the Zulu.' *Africa*, vol. 38, no. 29. pp. 173–200.

Kvale, S. 2001. *Det kvalitative forskningsintervju.* Oslo: Gyldendal Akademisk.

Laumann, E O & Gagnon, J H. 1995. 'A sociological perspective on sexual action.' In R G Parker & J H. Gagnon (eds). *Conceiving Sexuality: Approaches to Sex Research in a Postmodern World*, pp. 183–213. New York & London: Routledge.

LeClerc-Madlala, S. 2001a. 'Demonising women in the era of AIDS: On the relationship between cultural constructions of both HIV/AIDS and femininity.' *Society in Transition*, vol. 32, no. 1. pp. 38–46.

LeClerc-Madlala, S. 2001b. Virginity-testing: Managing sexuality in a maturing HIV/AIDS epidemic.' *Medical Anthropology Quarterly*, vol. 15, no. 4. pp. 533–52.

LeClerc-Madlala, S. 2002a. 'Youth, HIV/AIDS and the importance of sexual culture and context.' *Social Dynamics. Special Issue: AIDS and Society*, vol. 28, no. 1. pp. 20–41.

LeClerc-Madlala, S. 2002b. 'Prevention means more than condoms.' *Mail & Guardian Online*, 4–11 October.

Lemmer, E & Badenhorst, D. 1997. *Introduction to Education for South African Teachers: An Orientation of Teaching Practice*. Cape Town: Juta.

Levine, S & Ross, F. 2002. *Perceptions of and Attitudes to HIV/AIDS among Young Adults at the University of Cape Town*. Cape Town: Aids and Society Research Unit, Centre for Social Science Research, University of Cape Town. <http://web.uct.ac.za/depts/cssr/papers/wp14.pdf>. Accessed 8 January 2003.

Levine, S & Ross, F. 2002. 'Perceptions of and attitudes to HIV/AIDS among young adults in Cape Town.' *Social Dynamics: Special issue: AIDS and* Society, vol. 28, no. 1. pp. 89–108.

Louw, D. 1991. 'Ethics and Aids in the development structure.' In A. van Niekerk (ed.). *Aids in Context: A South African Perspective.* Cape Town: Lux Verbi.

loveLife. 2000. *Hot Prospects, Cold Facts: Portrait of Young South Africa*. Johannesburg: loveLife in conjunction with *The Sunday Times*.

Lugoe, W L & Klepp, K I. 1996. 'Sexual debut and predictors of condom use among secondary school students in Arusha, Tanzania.' *AIDS Care*, vol. 8, no. 4. pp. 443–52.

Mac an Ghail, M. 1996. *Understanding Masculinities: Social Relations and Cultural Arenas.* Buckingham: Open University Press.

Maharaj, P. 2001. 'Male attitudes to family planning in the era of HIV/AIDS: Evidence from KwaZulu-Natal, South Africa.' *Journal of Southern African Studies*, vol. 27, no. 2. pp. 246–57.

Mail & Guardian. 2003. 'AIDS activists lose patience with allies.' 13 January.

Mail & Guardian Online. 2008. 'At last, and end to lemons.' 20 October.

Makahye, G. 2005. 'Young men.' In S. S. A Karim & Q. A. Karim (eds). *HIV/AIDS in South Africa*, pp. 313–18. Cambridge: Cambridge University Press.

Makhate, M. 2002. 'An investigation into the perceptions of teachers and learners on HIV/AIDS in selected high schools in Mafeteng, Lesotho.' Unpublished honours dissertation, University of Cape Town.

Mamdani, M. 1996. *Citizen and Subject: Contemporary Africa and the Legacy of Late Colonialism*. Kampala: Fountain.

Mandela, N. 2002. *NHSRC Study of HIV/AIDS*. Household survey. Cape Town: NHSRC Press.

Marcus, T. 2000. 'Kissing the cobra: Sexuality and high risk in a generalised epidemic — a case study of white university students.' *African Journal of AIDS Research,* vol. 1, no. 1. pp. 23–39.

Mathews, C. 2005. 'Reducing sexual risk behaviours: Theory and research, successes and challenges.' In S. S. A Karim & Q. A. Karim (eds). *HIV/AIDS in South Africa*, pp. 143–65. Cambridge: Cambridge University Press.

Mbiti, J. 1969. *African Religions and Philosophy.* London, Ibadan & Nairobi: Heinemann.

Menka, E. 2005. *Science and Religion: Which should Lead the HIV/AIDS Prevention Campaign?* <http://www.ghanaweb.com/GhanaHomePage/features/artikel.php?ID=86656>. Accessed 30 March 2006.

Mirembe, R. 2002. 'AIDS and democratic education in Uganda.' *Comparative Education*, vol. 38, no. 3. pp. 291–303.

Morrell, R. 2001. 'The times of change: Men and masculinity in South Africa.' In R. Morrell (ed.). *Changing Men in Southern Africa*, pp. 3–40. Pietermaritzburg: University of Natal Press.

Muller, A & Steyn, M. 1999. 'Culture and the feasibility of a partnership between westernised medical practitioners and traditional healers.' *Society in Transition*, vol. 30, no. 2. pp. 142–57.

Muuss, R E. 1988. *Theories of Adolescence.* 5th ed. New York: McGraw-Hill.

Nagel, J. 2004. *Race, Ethnicity and Sexuality.* New York: Oxford University Press.

Nattrass, N. 2004. *The Moral Economy of AIDS in South Africa*. Cambridge: Cambridge University Press.

Netswera, F G. 2002. 'Risk awareness and sexual relationships among youth in the Johannesburg area.' *Health SA Gesondheid,* vol. 7, no. 3. pp. 79–88.

Ntshoe, I M. 1999. 'The impact of political violence on education in South Africa: Past, present and future.' *Current Issues in Comparative Education*, 2(1). <http://www.tc.columbia.edu/cice/vol02nr1/svart1.htm>. Accessed 1 October 2001.

Oster, E. 2007. *HIV and Sexual Behavior Change: Why not Africa?* National Bureau of Economic Research working paper. <http://ideas.repec.org/p/nbr/nberwo/13049.html>. Accessed 10 June 2008.

O'Sullivan, L F. et al 2006. 'Gender dynamics in the primary sexual relationships of young rural South African women and men.' In L. F. O'Sullivan et al (eds). *Culture, Health and Sexuality*. Publication information unavailable.

Ouzgane, L & Morrell, R. (eds). 2005. *African Masculinities: Men in Africa from the Late Nineteenth Century to the Present.* New York: Palgrave Macmillan.

Paasche-Orlow, S. & Rosenn, D. 2001. 'Judaism.' In R. A. Smith (ed.). *Encyclopedia of AIDS: A Social, Political, Cultural, and Scientific Record of the HIV Epidemic*, pp. 402–5. New York: Penguin.

Paquette, J. 1991. *Social Purpose and Schooling: Alternative Agendas and Issues.* London: Falmer Press.

Parker, R G & Gagnon, J. H. (eds). 1995. *Conceiving Sexuality: Approaches to Sex Research in a Postmodern World.* New York & London: Routledge.

Parker, S. 1995. 'Towards a theory of work and leisure.' In C. Critcher, P. Bramham & A. Tomlinson (eds). *Sociology of Leisure: A Reader*, pp. 261–65. London: E&Fn Spon.

Peltzer, K. et al 2005. *Educator Supply and Demand in the South African Public Education System: Integrated Report*. Pretoria: Human Sciences Research Council Press.

Pettifor, A E, Rees, H V, Steffenson, A, Hlongwa-Madikizela, L & MacPhail, C. 2004. *HIV and Sexual Behaviour among Young South Africans: A National Survey of 15–24 Year Olds.* Johannesburg: University of the Witwatersrand, Reproductive Health Research Unit.

Phillips, K M & Reay, B. (eds). 2002. *Sexualities in History: A Reader*. New York: Routledge.

Popkewitz, T S, Franklin, B M & Pereyra, M A. (eds). 2001. *Cultural History and Education: Critical Essays on Knowledge and Schooling.* New York: Routledge Falmer.

Prosser, J (ed.). 1999. *School Culture.* London: Paul Chapman.

Provincial Decision-making Enabling Project. 2005. 'A profile of the Western Cape province: Demographics, poverty, inequality and unemployment.' Background paper 2005:1(1). Elsenburg.

Reddy, S. 2003. 'Troubling sexualities: Young adults' sexual identity constructions within the context of HIV/AIDS.' Unpublished doctoral thesis, University of Durban-Westville.

Renold, E. 2000. '"Coming out": Gender, (hetero)sexuality and the primary school.' *Gender and Education*, vol. 12. pp. 309–26.

Rivers, K & Aggleton, P. 1999. *Adolescent Sexuality, Gender and the HIV Epidemic.* UNDP HIV and Development Programme. <http://www.undp.org/hiv/publications/gender/adolesce.htm>. Accessed 17 January 2003.

Rodgers, J L. 1996. 'Sexual transitions in adolescence.' In J. A. Graber et al (eds). *Transitions through Adolescence: Interpersonal Domains and Context*, pp. 85–110. New Jersey: Lawrence Erlbaum.

Rohmann, C. 2002. *The Dictionary of Important Ideas and Thinkers*. London: Arrow Books.

Sally, M. 1990. *Knowledge and Attitudes of a Group of Young People in Mitchells Plain Regarding Sexuality and AIDS*. Cape Town: University of Cape Town.

Sarason, S B. 1996. *Revisiting 'The Culture of the School and the Problem of Change'.* New York: Teachers College Press.

Schenker, I & Nyirenda, J M. 2002. *Preventing HIV/AIDS in Schools.* Brussels: International Academy of Education & Geneva: International Bureau of Education, UNESCO.

Seale, S. 2004. *Researching Society and Culture.* 2nd ed. London: Sage.

Simbayi, L C, Kalichman, S C, Jooste, S, Cherry, C, Mfecane, S & Cain, D. 2005. 'Risk factors for HIV/AIDS among youth in Cape Town, South Africa.' *AIDS and Behaviour,* vol. 9, no. 1. pp. 53–61.

Simbayi, L C, Skinner, D., Letlape, L. & Zuma, K. 2005. *Workplace Policies in Public Education: A Review Focusing on HIV/AIDS*. Cape Town: Human Sciences Research Council Press.

Simon, W & Gagnon, J H. 1987. 'A sexual scripts approach.' In J. H. Geer & W. T. O'Donohue (eds). *Theories of Human Sexuality: Perspectives in Sexuality: Behavior, Research and Therapy*, pp. 363–84. New York & London: Plenum Press.

Skinner, D. 2000. 'A practical application of psychological theory: Use of the theories of reasoned action and planned behaviour to gain a better understanding of HIV related behavior among youth in the communities of Kayamandi and Mbekweni.' Unpublished doctoral thesis, University of Cape Town.

Skinner, D. 2001. *How Do the Youth in Two Communities Make Decisions about Using Condoms?* Cape Town: Aids and Society Research Unit, Centre for Social Science Research, University of Cape Town. <http://web.uct.ac.za/depts/cssr/papers/wp2.pdf>. Accessed 1 September 2003.

Skinner, D & Mfecane, S. 2004. 'Stigma and discrimination and the implications for people living with HIV/AIDS in South Africa.' *Journal of Social Aspects of HIV/AIDS*, vol. 1, no. 3. pp. 157–64.

Smith, R A. 2001. *Encyclopedia of AIDS: A Social, Political, Cultural, and Scientific Record of the HIV Epidemic.* New York: Penguin.

Smith, L C, Lucas, K J & Latkin, C. 1999. 'Rumor and gossip: Social discourse on HIV and AIDS.' *Anthropology and Medicine*, vol. 6, no. 1. pp. 121–31.

Sobo, E J. 1995. *Choosing Unsafe Sex: AIDS-risk Denial among Disadvantaged Women.* Philadelphia: University of Pennsylvania Press.

Sogolo, G. 1995. 'African philosophy and social science research in contemporary Africa.' Discussion paper presented at the Human Sciences Research Council, Pretoria, 25 October.

Sontag, S. 1990. *AIDS and Its Metaphors*. London: Penguin.

South Africa. 1999. 'National policy on HIV/AIDS for learners and educators in public schools, and students and educators.' *Government Gazette*, 20372.

South Africa. 2000. *HIV/Aids/STD Strategic Plan for South Africa 2000–2005*. Pretoria. <http://www.info.gov.za/otherdocs/2000/aidsplan2000.pdf>. Accessed 17 December 2004.

South Africa.info. 2005. *HIV/AIDS in South Africa.* <http://www.southafrica.info/ess_info/sa_glance/health/aids.htm>. Accessed 1 March 2005.

South Africa.info. 2007. *Health Care in South Africa*. <http://www.southafrica.info/ess_info/sa_glance/health/AIDS.htm>. Accessed 15 July 2007

Stadler, J. 2001. *Looking at loveLife: The First Year: Summaries of Monitoring and Evaluation*. <http://www.kff.org/docs/sections/safrica/firstyear_report.pdf>. Accessed 13 January 2003.

Steinberg, J. 2008. *Sizwe's Test: A Young Man's Journey Through Africa's Aids Epidemic*. New York, London, Toronto & Sydney: Simon & Schuster.

Steinberg, M, Johnson, S, Schierhout, G & Ndegwa, D. 2002. 'Hitting home: How households cope with the impact of the HIV/AIDS epidemic: A survey of households affected by HIV/AIDS in South Africa.' Durban: Health Systems Trust.

Susser, I & Stein, Z. 2000. 'Culture, sexuality, and women's agency in the prevention of HIV/AIDS in Southern Africa.' *American Journal of Public Health*, vol. 90, no. 7. pp. 1042–53.

Swartz, D. 1997. *Culture and Power: The Sociology of Pierre Bourdieu.* Chicago: University of Chicago Press.

Thanvi, A A. 1992. *Etiquettes of Social Life*. New Delhi: Idara Ishaat-e-dinitat.

Tillotson, J & Maharaj, P. 2001. 'Barriers to HIV/AIDS protective behaviour among African adolescent males in township secondary schools in Durban, South Africa.' *Society in Transition*, vol. 32, no. 1. pp. 83–100.

UNAIDS (Joint UN Action Plan on HIV/AIDS). 2000. *International Partnership against AIDS in Africa*. Geneva: UNAIDS.

UNAIDS (Joint UN Action Plan on HIV/AIDS). 2005. *Aids Epidemic Update*. Geneva: UNAIDS.

UNAIDS (Joint UN Action Plan on HIV/AIDS). 2006a. *Report on the Global AIDS Epidemic*. New York: UNAIDS. <http://www.unaids.org/en/KnowledgeCentre/HIVData/GlobalReport/Default.asp>. Accessed 10 June 2008.

UNAIDS (Joint UN Action Plan on HIV/AIDS). 2006b. *Uniting the world against AIDS*. <http://www.unaids.org/en/Regions_Countries/south_africa.asp>. Accessed 25 March 2006.

University of Texas. 2005. *Understanding School Culture.* <http://wings.utexas.org/school-culture.html>. Accessed 5 May 2005.

Van Wijk, B. 1994. 'The dynamics of HIV transmission amongst a group of school-going adolescents in South Africa.' Unpublished honours dissertation, University of Cape Town.

Varga, C. 1997. 'Sexual decision-making and negotiation in the midst of AIDS: Youth in KwaZulu-Natal, South Africa.' *Health Transition Review (Supplement)*, vol. 3, no. 7. pp. 45–47.

Walker, L, Reid, G & Cornell, M. 2004. *Waiting to Happen: HIV/AIDS in South Africa: The Bigger Picture*. Boulder: Lynne Rienner.

Wallis, A & VanEvery, J. 2000. 'Sexuality in the primary school.' *Sexualities*, vol. 3, no. 4. pp. 409–24.

Wangenge-Ouma, G. 2007. 'Trap of death: How village life exposes Kenyan youth to HIV/AIDS.' In H. Charton & C. Medard (eds). *L'Afrique Orientale: Annuaire 2005*, pp. 271–97. Paris: L'Harmattan.

WCED (Western Cape Education Department). 2002. *WCED: HIV/AIDS Lifeskills Programme*. <http//wced.wcape.gov.za/planning&devel/support/special_ed/hiv_aids/info_ 2003.html>. Accessed 3 March 2005.

Weeks, J. 2002. 'Sexuality and history revisited.' In K. M. Phillips & B. Reay (eds). *Sexualities in History: A Reader*, pp. 27–41. New York: Routledge.

Wight, D. 1999. 'Limits to empowerment-based sex education.' *Health Education,* vol. 99, no. 6. pp. 233–43.

Wood, K & Jewkes, R. 1997a. *'Love Is a Dangerous Thing': Micro-dynamics of Violence in Sexual Relationships of Young People in Umtata*. Medical Research Council. <http://www.mrc.ac.za/researchreports/finallove.pdf>. Accessed 17 January 2003.

Wood, K & Jewkes, R. 1997b. 'Violence, rape, and sexual coercion: Everyday love in a South African township.' *Gender and Development: Men and Masculinity,* vol. 5, no. 2. pp. 41–46.

Wood, K & Jewkes, R. 1998. 'He forced me to love him: Putting violence on adolescents' sexual health agendas.' *Social Science and Medicine,* vol. 47, no. 2. pp. 233–42.

Wood, K & Jewkes, R. 2001. '"Dangerous" love: Reflections on violence among Xhosa township youth.' In R. Morrell (ed.). *Changing Men in Southern Africa*, pp. 317–36. Pietermaritzburg: University of Natal Press.

Wood, K, Maepa, J & Jewkes, R. 1997. *Adolescent Sex and Contraceptive Experiences: Perspectives of Teenagers and Clinic Nurses in the Northern Province*. Medical Research Council. <http://www.mrc.ac.za/researchreports/contra.pdf>.

World Bank. 2000. *Exploring the Implications of the HIV/AIDS Epidemic for Educational Planning in Selected African Countries: The Demographic Question.* ACTafrica, AIDS Campaign Team for Africa. Washington, DC: World Bank.

Wyner, N (ed.). 1991. *Current Perspectives on the Culture of Schools.* Cambridge, Mass.: Brookline Books.

Yamauchi, L A & O'Donnell, C R. 2005. 'Considering the context of behavior change.' In C R O'Donnell & L A Yamauchi (eds). *Culture and Context in Human Behavior Change*, pp. 3–12. New York: Peter Lang.

Index

L

M

N

R